THRIVING
WITH
RHEUMATOID ARTHRITIS

Diana Girnita MD, PhD

Copyright © 2024 by Diana Girnita

All rights are reserved, and no part of this publication may be reproduced, distributed, or transmitted in any manner, whether through photocopying, recording, or any other electronic or mechanical methods, without the explicit prior written permission of the publisher. This restriction applies to any form or means of reproduction or distribution.

Exceptions to this rule include brief quotations that may be incorporated into critical reviews, as well as certain other noncommercial uses that are allowed by copyright law. Any such usage must adhere to the specified conditions and permissions outlined by the copyright holder.

ISBN: 979-8-218-49965-5

Disclaimer

This book is intended as a general guide only and should never be a substitute for the expertise of a qualified medical professional who can address the unique facts, circumstances, and symptoms of an individual case. The nutritional, medical, and health information provided is based on the research, training, and professional experience of the author and is true and complete to the best of her knowledge. However, this book is for informational purposes only and is not intended to replace medical advice from a healthcare provider. Each person and each situation is unique, and you should consult a professional trainer before engaging in any physical exercise.

The author and publisher are not responsible for any adverse effects or consequences resulting from the application of information presented in this book. It is your responsibility to discuss any health concerns with your healthcare provider. The recipes included in this book were chosen by the author based on her preferences. If you have food allergies or sensitivities, avoid any recipes with ingredients that may cause a reaction. All recipes are used at the risk of the consumer, and the author assumes no responsibility for any hazards, loss, or damage that may result from their use.

At the time of publication, all referenced URLs link to active websites. Dr. Girnita is not responsible for maintaining and does not endorse content not created by her.

Advance Praise for "THRIVING WITH RHEUMATOID ARTHRITIS"

"A step-by-step guide that's life changing for RA."

Will Bulsiewicz, MD MSCI
New York Times bestselling author

"In the avalanche of medical information that patients and healthcare providers face, Dr. Diana Girnita's book *Thriving with Rheumatoid Arthritis* brings much-needed clarity to holistic care. It is a powerful testimonial of what Integrative Medicine offers in Rheumatology.

Backed by the latest medical science and with a compelling but honest voice, Dr Girnita empowers patients to learn, heal, and ultimately thrive while living with RA. Dr. Girnita's extensive training in immunology, rheumatology, lifestyle medicine, and nutrition is at the forefront of this practical, actionable, and motivational patient guide. Each story shared provides the sense that the physician, Dr. Girnita, is being changed along with her patients. With the simplicity that accompanies subject mastery and the humility of a true healer, Dr. Girnita provides "prescriptions" on nutrition, sleep, exercise, stress management, self-compassion, and self-care.

The book goes way beyond the promise of its title. Dr. Girnita's teachings provide a humanistic and supportive environment for healing and creating a purposeful and beautiful journey while living with RA.

You can sense her out-cry to better our medical system, specifically highlighting its focus on "sick care" rather than genuine "health care" for prevention rather than intervention.

In my quest to promote Integrative Medicine, I look forward to recommending this book to patients and colleagues alike for its clear and hopeful depiction of holistic care in Rheumatology."

Mihaela Taylor, MD,
Professor of Clinical Medicine, UCLA David Geffen School of Medicine

"Thriving with Rheumatoid Arthritis" is a comprehensive, scientifically sound and relatable journey for the reader to know what it is like to have a devasting disease such as rheumatoid arthritis (RA). Dr. Girnita's brutal honesty about the current state of our country's health care system and how it is failing our patients is heartbreaking for health care professionals to admit (but also very true!). Fortunately, she has developed an exciting holistic approach to care that involves patients in shared decision making and empowers her patients to have a voice and the ability to control this painful and debilitating disease. Through many different methods, both traditional and novel, the reader learns what he/she can do to live a healthy, productive life while also living with RA. Congratulations, Dr. Girnita. This book is a triumph for all of us, patients and caregivers alike, who are searching for another way to approach wellness.

Avis Ware, MD
Professor of Clinical; Rheumatology Division Chief;
University of Cincinnati Medical College

My experience reading Thriving with Rheumatoid Arthritis, by Diana Girnita MD, PhD, was like being in a living room and having a long conversation with a close friend. Dr. Girnita greets us and proceeds to nourish the reader with new knowledge and wise advice. In a conversational, non-stuffy tone, she teaches science, empathizes with the challenge of living with the painful and debilitating chronic illness, rheumatoid arthritis (RA), and provides comprehensive and practical advice about treatment. I felt right in the room with her as she has a dialogue with her patients, putting herself in their position, using many helpful stories and anecdotes which help the reader understand and brings the content alive. She encourages the patient to be the "CEO of their RA" and shows there is so much more than medications alone which can help disease management. She provides in depth insight about the value of exercise, diet, mindfulness, meditation, stress reduction and a host of other self-management approaches, summarizing research as well as providing lived experience. I especially appreciated the section of her book devoted to the importance of relationships with others. For many people, having a chronic illness like RA is not only physically impactful but can cause a person to go inward and be alienated from friends and family. Combating feelings of depression and loneliness is a crucial part of healthy living. Although I think this book will be most helpful for patients and their loved ones, it is also a useful compendium for health care practitioners. I have thought of myself as reasonably knowledgeable about RA and a relatively good medical communicator for my patients, but was humbled by the breadth and depth of insights that Dr. Girnita brings to the conversation with patients that are with her. We are grateful that this book allows us to learn from this conversation.

Philip Mease MD, MACR;
Director, Rheumatology Research, Providence Swedish Health and Director,
Seattle Rheumatology Associates, Seattle, WA, USA

THANK YOU

A few years ago, I unexpectedly lost my mother. Her passing left an incredible mark on my heart. My mom was a beacon of compassion, dedicating her life to her children, grandchildren, family, and friends.

Mom, you were an inspiration to me! I still remember how you always encouraged me to eat healthily and take care of myself. I am sure you're smiling down on us from above, happy for all we've accomplished.

I want to thank my father, whose unwavering, quiet kindness and support have been a constant source of strength during challenging times.

A big hug and thank you to my children Ana, Alysa, and Edi. You have been an incredible source of support through your patience during the times I worked tremendously to grow my practice, Rheumatologist OnCall. Your love has been my driving force!

I'm profoundly thankful for my brother, who has been an unwavering cheerleader for my work. His encouragement during dark moments and his belief in my innovative approach to telemedicine pushed me to continue on this path, allowing me to help patients worldwide.

To the friends, mentors and my colleagues who believed in me and offered their support along the way, I extend my heartfelt gratitude. A special "Thank you" to Cori Gramescu that dedicated her time and shared the pictures with exercises in this book.

Most importantly, I am grateful to my patients, whose real stories form the heart of this book. They have been, and continue to be, my greatest teachers. Every day, they push me to expand my knowledge and challenge the boundaries of conventional Western medicine. Their trust in my ability to heal and help, even from hundreds or thousands of miles away, has been profoundly humbling and motivating. My patients inspired me to delve deeper into scientific research, exploring the powerful intersection of nutrition, lifestyle changes, and evidence-based medicine. Their experiences and our shared journey of healing have shaped not only this book but also my entire approach to medical care.

This book is a testament to the power of family, friendship, patient trust, and perseverance. It stands as a tribute to those who are no longer with me, those who stand beside me, and the enduring spirit of compassion and innovation through telemedicine in medical care.

This book is a celebration of the incredible lessons learned from my patients who dared to believe in the possibility of healing across great distances.

With deepest appreciation,
DR. G

Contents

Author's Note 13
   Patients taught me the missing link in medical care 17
   From sick care to true healthcare.. 19

01. Cut Through the Noise: Guidance for Rheumatoid Arthritis 23
   What is Rheumatoid Arthritis? 26
   Beyond the Prescription Pad: Why Lifestyle Matters.. 27
   Google Isn't Your Doctor 30

02. Understanding the Past to Improve the Present.. 33
   Then and Now: The History of RA. 35
   Famous Faces of RA: Those Who Share the Struggle.. 37

03. Rheumatoid Arthritis 101 41
   Why Me? Who is Affected By RA?.. 44
   RA Day-to-Day: What to Expect 48
      Which Symptoms Should I Expect? 49
      What About the UNCOMMON Signs and Symptoms of RA? .. 50
   How Is RA Diagnosed? 51
      The Journey to Diagnosis 52
      What Are the Most Common Imaging Tests for RA? 54
      The Dangers of Google 56
   How Is RA Treated? The Old, New, and Future 57
      Living Without Treatment: What Can Go Wrong?. 58
      Current Treatments: What's Out There? 62
   What *Isn't* RA? 69
      Gout and RA 70
      RA vs Lupus.. 71
      RA vs. Psoriatic Arthritis 72
      RA vs. Sjogren's 72
   Hope For Your Future 73

04. Trust Your Gut 75
   Humans Don't Run the World—Bugs Do 77
      The Microbial 'Engine'. 78
      The Body's Second Immune System 79
      Living In Harmony: The Impact of Microbial Dysbiosis 81
   Go With Your Gut: RA, Dysbiosis, and the Gut Microbiome 83
   It All Comes Back To Lifestyle.. 85

05. Nutrition 101: Detoxify, Heal, and Supercharge 87

Detoxification 101 90
- Sugar. 90
- High Fructose Corn Syrup (HFCS) 93
- Sugar & Rheumatoid arthritis 94
- Salt. 96
- Fats & Oils: The Good and The Bad 96
- Dairy. 99
- Gluten.. 101
- Nightshade Vegetables.. 103
- Coffee 105
- After Elimination: What's Next? 106

Healing Your Body 101 107
- Healing Your Gut with More Fiber. 107
- The More Fiber, the More SCFAs 109
- Without Fiber, What Happens? 110
- Where can you get fiber? 111
- Whole Grains 111
- Fruits 113
- Green Vegetables 116
- Legumes.. 118
- Nuts and Seeds. 121
- Probiotics 124
- Prebiotics 125
- Healthy Fats.. 126
- Spice Up Your Food 128
- Green Tea 131

Supercharge 101 RA-friendly Diets. 132
- The Mediterranean Diet.. 132
- A Vegan Diet. 135
- The RA-Friendly Food Pyramid 137

Reclaiming Your Future: Diet and RA 139

06. The Not-So Bitter Pills 141

Supplements 101 143
- Fish Oil & Omega-3s 146
- Turmeric 148
- Probiotics 149
- Vitamin D.. 150
- Other Supplements That Fight RA Symptoms 152

Get Started with Supplements 154

07. It's Not In Your Head: Stress, RA, and Healing **157**
    The Mind-Body Connection.. 160
    A Vicious Cycle: Stress & the Immune System 161
    Does Stress Cause RA?.. 163
    Stress & RA: The Last Piece of the Puzzle 164
    Fight the Stress 165
    Mindfulness: A Key Stress-busting Intervention 166
    Mindfulness & Medicine: Does It Actually Work? 166
    Your Mindfulness Journey: The Beginning.. 171
    Ommm, Ommm: Reclaim Your Body with Meditation 173
    How to Practice Meditation? 175
    Breathing Better 177
    Shift Your Mindset: Healthy Stress-Reduction Practices 180
        Quit the Complaining Habit 180
        Say "Thank You": Gratitude and RA 181
        Live in the Happy Moments 183
    Your Stress-Free Journey 184

08. Motion is Lotion: How to Get Movin' **187**
    What Are The Benefits of Exercise?. 189
    Exercise & RA: Motion is Lotion For Your Joints 190
    How to Get Movin' 191
    Aquatic Therapy 194
    Keep On Movin' 197

09. Get Some Rest: Sleep & RA **199**
    What Is Sleep? 201
    Why Is Sleep So Important For Those With RA? 202
    How Can You Improve Your Sleep? 205
    Get Started With Better Sleep 207

10. Natural Remedies That Work (And Those That *Don't*) **209**
    Natural Remedies That Don't Work 213
        Magnet Therapy.. 213
        Copper Bracelets 213
        Fish Tank Therapy.. 214
        Ozone Therapy. 214
        Cherry Juice 214

  Glucosamine and Collagen Supplements. 215
  Bee Venom. 215
  Just Say 'No' to Remedies That Don't Work 215
 Natural Remedies That Work. 216
  Vagus Nerve Stimulation. 216
  Salt Baths 217
  Paraffin Wax Bath 217
  Manuka Honey 217
  Melatonin 218
  Sauna 218
  CBD Oil or Cream 218

11. The Power of Community 223
 Loneliness On the Rise 225
 Stay Connected: RA & Loneliness 226
 Release Yourself From the Loneliness Trap 228
 Get Connected 229

12. Become the CEO of Your RA. 231
 RA and Your Health-Related Quality of Life.. 234
 The Blue Zone Lifestyle: Coming Full Circle. 234
 Reclaim Your Future With RA.. 237

References. 239
Patient Resources 257

AUTHOR'S NOTE

When patients seek care and contact a medical group, they're typically assigned a physician on the spot based on basic information they share when they call for the first time. The patient is given a name, a time, and a date, leaving them with little information about the person who will take care of their most profound, and sometimes most intimate, concerns for months or years to come. Once they have this information, many patients consult Google, and find the doctor's professional bio, which details their training and academic background. Most bios, mine included, don't answer the patient's most pressing question—*can this person help me? Will this person make me feel seen and understood?*

When patients finally visit the office for their first appointment, they're asked many probing questions about their background and medical history. A nurse, and later a doctor, ask about their habits, past, and present—*what brings you in today? Do you smoke? What about family history?* These questions, too, feel insufficient, dancing around the truth about why most people go to the doctor: They're in pain.

The vibe in most medical offices is cold. Seldom, if ever, do most offices have windows or brightly colored posters, and the fluorescent lighting casts an unsympathetic glare over the intimate conversations happening inside. These conversations, particularly during a first appointment, feel more like a business meeting than a conversation about what's genuinely plaguing a patient. Sensitivity is utterly absent, creating a lopsided balance of vulnerability between the patient and their doctor: I, the doctor, leave knowing all of their intimate details, their history, and their pain. The patient leaves knowing little about their physician, the person responsible for their care. I sought to change this in my practice, Rheumatologist OnCall.

So, in this section, I aim to be vulnerable and honest with you, telling you why I sought to change traditional medicine in my practice, Rheumatologist OnCall, and how the changes I made continue to help those like you who have been diagnosed with Rheumatoid arthritis. I will share many stories in this book with you, but I'd like to start with my own now.

I was born and raised in Romania, an eastern European country of less than twenty million people. I grew up in Craiova, a relatively tightly-knit city.

Twelve-year-olds are supposed to be filled with joy and energy, but I was anything but—I was exhausted all the time and had grown jaundiced over just a few days. My skin and eyes were a bright yellow color, and my mother, the caring, observant woman she is, grew alarmed.

I remember her taking me to the doctor. He examined me and told my mother that I needed to be admitted—immediately. So, for the first time in my short life, I was admitted to the hospital. And soon, after numerous pokes and prods and uncomfortable conversations, I learned my symptoms were indicative of a mysterious liver disease. I overheard one of the doctors say, "Her immune system is fighting her body and attacking her liver," which struck fear into my heart. Even at my young age, I understood that, if left untreated, the disease would destroy my liver. I knew this was a critical, life-threatening situation.

To this day, I vividly remember the doctor who took care of me during my hospitalization. He was compassionate, speaking to me only in words he knew I could understand. As he was treating me, he explained what he was doing, why he was doing it, and how it would potentially help me. He touched my forehead to reassure me and lightly scolded me, saying, "You need to eat your fruits today!" "How did you sleep last night?" or, "Did you smile today?" I found all of this incredibly reassuring, and these expressions of genuine concern stayed with me long after I was discharged. It was a challenging journey, but with the help of treatment, proper nutrition, and rest, I recovered from my illness after about a year.

That experience changed my life forever, sparking my desire to become a physician. At age fifteen, I made up my mind: I would make my dream a reality. I became my family's first college graduate and, six years later, the first to graduate from medical school.

Standing where I am now, with twenty years of experience and an ongoing medical practice, and looking back on those early days, it feels like it went by instantly. But rest assured, I enjoyed every step along the way. I was passionate about learning and discovering, and I loved teaching those around me about the little things I was learning to enhance their medical knowledge.

After medical school, I began my career as a cardiology resident in Romania, where I stayed for about three years. However, I developed a passion for the immune system and genetics and how both intertwine with overall health. So, I decided to deepen my understanding by returning to school and pursuing a doctorate degree (Ph.D.) in medicine.

Although I'd worked hard to get admitted into a Ph.D. program, it was still a surprise when, while I was still working on this additional advanced degree, I was invited to publish and present at local and European conferences. I had very few resources and seemingly no connections when these invitations came. In Romania, like in many other countries, it's all about connections; being the son or daughter of another doctor opens many doors. But my parents were hard-working lower middle-class people from Romania. Although they supported my ambitions, it was up to me to break boundaries and find opportunities to grow in a field that sometimes can be hostile if you aren't part of the chosen "team" or friends with the "right" people.

After completing my Ph.D., I began applying to U.S. universities to complete a postdoctoral fellowship. In 2004, after many applications, I was finally invited to Harvard University! Initially, I thought this couldn't be true! Until I arrived in Boston, I often felt something would happen out of thin air or that it was a mistake, and I wouldn't be able to honor the invitation.

To make my trip a reality, my parents sold a piece of land and put $2,000 in my hands. A friend borrowed money so that I could pay for the flight. I felt honored and indebted to them for their generosity and for believing in my future.

On January 5th, 2005, I took an airplane for the first time. After a 15-hour flight, I stepped onto American soil with one suitcase filled with medical books and a few pieces of clothing. Though I had finished medical school and was a practicing doctor, I still saw myself as a simple girl from a small country. And here I was, coming to the land of over 300 million people, hoping to find knowledge, exploration, and research. It was surreal. I had never dreamed of coming to America, much less to a prestigious institution like Harvard University.

In Boston, I lived a life that I couldn't have imagined when I was a young, sick, 12-year-old girl. While the $2,000 was barely enough to cover my deposit, first month's rent, and food for a few weeks, I felt full of hope. In Romania, my salary was $79 a month, but I was paid $2,000 a month in the

United States. My rent was $1,200 monthly, and utilities were around $300, but I felt rich with $500 left to live. My studio was in a basement, but I felt fortunate to live near the medical center where I worked. When I went to Harvard Medical School for the first time and saw the ornate library featuring medical instruments used throughout history, I felt so emotional. I could see what I'd dreamed of and read books about for the first time in person.

I was fortunate to attend seminars by famous physicians like Dr. Eugene Braunwald, a prestigious cardiologist and a distinguished Professor of Medicine at Harvard Medical School. I also saw Dr. James Watson, who, with Francis Crick, discovered the famous DNA double helix, which won the two of them the Nobel Prize, speak. I cried seeing them in person. In Romania, my parents had spent nearly both their salaries buying me Dr. Braunwald's cardiology textbooks. Attending lectures by these incredible scientists solidified my path—I'd made the right choice.

Little did I know that after just a year in the U.S., I would move to the University of Pittsburgh to work as a postdoctoral associate at the Thomas Starzl Institute, the world's largest transplant center at that time. There, I personally met one of the titans of Immunology, Dr. Thomas Starzl, the surgeon who did the world's first successful liver transplant. I attended many of his lectures and seminars, and I felt fortunate to work and coordinate a project involving six of the world's largest transplant centers. I coordinated a multicenter grant alongside physicians at Columbia University, Stanford University, Pittsburgh, Loma Linda, and Washington University. I studied the genetics of different molecules influencing inflammation and rejection rates in children receiving heart transplants. This study helped us understand how genetics can impact our immune system. My research showed that genetics significantly affects whether a heart transplant is accepted or rejected.

After much work, our results positively impacted the lives of thousands of people, including children in need of heart transplants. During this time, I had the pleasure of presenting many times at the American Transplant Congress, the largest conference on transplantation in the world.

However, in my stomach was a nagging feeling that wouldn't disappear—something was missing. After five long years of successful clinical research, I missed patient interactions. After all, patients like myself inspired me to go into medicine. I wanted to help them. Today, years later, patients are still my primary motivation, fueling me each day and driving me to continue learning and coming to work each morning. So, I decided to take the plunge once again and undergo further training to become board-certified in Internal Medicine and Rheumatology. Why Rheumatology? And let me tell you—it was worth it.

After two years of preparing, taking multiple exams, interviewing, three years of residency, and another two years of fellowship, I finally found myself in rheumatology, a dynamic field in which doctors manage and treat chronic inflammation, the root cause of some of the most devastating diseases plaguing humans. I was proud to be in a booming field wrought with scientific advancements; research in rheumatology was, and is, still in its infancy. New treatments for autoimmune diseases such as Rheumatoid arthritis and Psoriatic Arthritis are released every few years. I was excited to learn even more about our immune system and to make a huge difference in patients' lives.

Patients taught me the missing link in medical care

When I first started practicing, I genuinely thought I had to treat my patients–all of the targeted therapies I had learned about were supposed to work. It didn't take long before I had evaluated thousands of patients with autoimmune diseases, many with rheumatoid arthritis (a condition I became very passionate about): Within the first three years, I realized that while some of my patients respond well to new, targeted therapies, too many do not. Only 60% of our Rheumatoid arthritis patients react to even the most advanced scientific, cutting-edge treatments. Researchers believe they've stumbled upon a miracle treatment, only for it to work on just some patients—not all.

Somehow, through interactions I couldn't yet name, I started to see more and more patients with Rheumatoid arthritis (we'll use the standard abbreviation RA many times in this book). I was fascinated by their stories, many of which you'll read in this book. My patient's stories led me to wonder, *Was I truly offering them the best care possible? How could I better assist them in managing their inflammation and pain, ensuring they led more fulfilling lives?*

I decided to interview my patients, and the revelations in these conversations were nothing short of astonishing. The patients I spoke with

with who were most successful at managing their RA assured me that, while their clinical medications helped, it wasn't the medication alone that truly prompted their healing process: Those patients with positive outcomes, who were free of disability and pain, spoke extensively about dietary changes they'd made: meditation, mindfulness, exercise, and the support of their loved ones, in addition to medication when necessary. These lifestyle changes compelled their healing, not the medications I'd come to rely on as a physician. As you read, you'll uncover the full scope of these findings, and I hope you, too, can use these to find relief from this disease.

Oddly enough, for a profession so rooted in health, we physicians are left in the dark about the profound effects of lifestyle on a patient's well-being. Most physicians, including myself, only spend about four hours in their 10 years of total medical training discussing or learning about the food we eat and its impact on our health. Read that again: Four hours discussing nutrition and its impact in 10 years of study. Other topics, like meditation and mindfulness, are discussed even less. It's no wonder we physicians often dismiss them.

I decided I wasn't going to be one of those physicians. After my last fellowship, I thought I was finished with my medical training. I couldn't have been more wrong—just three years after graduating from my fellowship program and after interviewing my patients, I returned to school, studying Nutrition Science at Stanford University and Mindfulness at the University of Massachusetts. I spent hundreds of thousands of hours researching all of the topics I'll explain and discuss in this book.

My patient's stories led me to introspection: Was I truly offering them the best care possible? How could I better assist them in managing their inflammation and pain, ensuring they led more fulfilling lives?

I shared with my patients what I learned, and they started to apply these scientifically proven strategies. Within months, many returned to express their gratitude: They weren't just following dietary advice but integrating science into their daily lives. The evidence was clear—my approach was working. They reported renewed energy, reduced pain, and increased flexibility.

Many even found themselves relying less on medication! Remarkably, these transformative changes unfolded in mere weeks.

From sick care to true healthcare

As discussed earlier in this section, working in a traditional medical practice has its difficulties. Most physicians, including myself, at times, don't have much control over the stark clinical environments in which we're supposed to practice. These environments, coupled with the cold, impersonal questions we're taught to ask patients, do little to put them at ease, making them feel like they're at the Department of Motor Vehicles discussing documentation, not answering intimate questions about how they truly feel.

> *We've inadvertently built an approach centered on "sick care" rather than genuine medical care.*

Traditional practice only allows physicians a certain amount of time with each patient, usually under 15 minutes (sometimes less). Many physicians face the paradox of being penalized for spending "extra" time with patients: Surprisingly (or not), physician compensation often hinges on productivity metrics rather than the quality of patient care they provide. Unfortunately, because of the constraints placed on us by traditional practice, most physicians don't have the time to educate patients about the intricate components of their disease. In other words, the goal is more patients, which equates to more revenue, causing doctors to gloss over potentially essential elements of a patient's disease or treatment plan.

This approach aligns more with treating symptoms than fostering genuine, overall health. Rather than addressing a patient's underlying issues, our primary approach is treating pain, using medications—often expensive ones—to mask or alleviate symptoms. When one drug falls short, another drug is proposed as an option to try. Unfortunately, if a solution isn't found, blame shifts to the patients themselves: They may be labeled as noncompliant, overly vocal about their concerns, or even told it's "all in their heads."

Plus, the traditional medical system doesn't incentivize physicians who discuss preventative or non-prescription healing measures with patients. For years, while practicing in a traditional setting, I was strongly motivated to provide the best medical care possible to everyone who came to my practice, but I lacked the time. Even when I struggled to give my patients more information, I knew they couldn't access me until their next appointment, often many months away. How much could I tell them and expect them to remember? What should I address with each patient first in the seven to 15 minutes I had with them? Should I listen to their symptoms, write orders, struggle to jot down notes, think about what billing codes to enter, or educate patients about nutrition and other lifestyle interventions? I was clear about the approach I wanted to take, but it also haunted me. I simply didn't have enough time for all I wanted to do for them.

Navigating the constraints of a traditional medical practice proved challenging. Despite my sincere commitment to providing top-tier care, the time constraints placed on my shoulders left me feeling inadequate. Even on occasions when I managed to share vital information, follow-up consultations were spaced out by months at a time, limiting continuous care and guidance.

What I (and my patients) were experiencing cuts to the heart of the hardest part of practicing medicine today: We have a healthcare system that's great at identifying problems but horrible at truly solving them. I wondered, "If our aim becomes prevention and holistic well-being, who remains for the system to treat?" The healthcare system's priority felt monetary rather than helping patients feel better. I understood that medical care didn't equate to "healthcare" as promoted by hospital-owned practices.

We've inadvertently built an approach centered on *"sick care"* rather than *genuine medical care.* Thus, I chose to step away from traditional practice, forging a path and creating my own clinic.

In my own private practice, I determine the rhythm of patient appointments, serving as a physician, lifestyle coach, and healer. I had to learn to both use science to understand and accept Mother Nature's role in influencing our immune system. My practices' unique approach melds lifestyle medicine with traditional practices, harnessing the pinnacle of my combined expertise to empower those with RA to thrive rather than merely survive.

My journey hasn't been easy, but it has been unforgettable. I am grateful for every challenge that has shaped me into the physician and researcher I am today.

If you're here, reading this book, you are ready to immerse yourself in your own journey. Dive deep into the effects of various medications, the immune system, inflammation, autoimmune diseases, gut health, nutrition, sleep, stress, and exercise. Learn about the history of Rheumatoid arthritis and how its appearance in a patient's life often has no rhyme or reason. Here, I'll teach you how to make sure you feed your gut microbiome to keep it happy, and how this translates into better control of your symptoms. Together, we'll craft a nutrition plan steeped in anti-inflammatory principles to discover which foods exacerbate inflammation and which act as its antidote. It's a lifestyle, not a diet—and because no diet is sustainable, your lifestyle will shape your healthy future and allow you to use as little prescription medicine as possible.

The information in this book is a collection of everything I've learned, studied, read, and practiced over the last twenty years. While this book chronicles my experiences with patients, the different types of pharmaceuticals I recommend, the lifestyle changes I suggest, and my patients' journeys, it also paves the way for your own transformative experience.

CHAPTER 1

CUT THROUGH THE NOISE: GUIDANCE FOR RHEUMATOID ARTHRITIS

When Georgia[1] came to see me, she was 42—at the prime of her life. She was her family's breadwinner and the owner of a successful baking company. I'd been familiar with her famous cannolis long before she came into my office. When she entered my office, I immediately noticed her hunched posture–Georgia walked like someone much older than her, bent over and moaning with each step.

"Doc, I've always been healthy, but I've never been in so much pain," she told me. Georgia explained that, over only four weeks, she had developed a deep pain and swelling in her wrists and elbows that prevented her from working. Then, in the two weeks before our appointment, she developed swelling in both of her knees and found herself barely able to walk.

"I went to the urgent care center, and they sent me to the emergency room. The pills they gave me barely touched the pain. And they didn't even tell me what I have!"

Based on the symptoms she described, I knew that Georgia's diagnosis was likely RA. And, like so many of my RA patients, her physical symptoms were accompanied by a chaotic and confused emotional state. I knew that she needed help, even though she didn't ask me for it explicitly.

"Georgia, I am here to help you," I told her. "You and I will be partners on this journey. I will help you improve, and you must trust me." I assisted Georgia to the examining table and examined her wrists, elbows, and knees. I began discussing with Georgia the steps we would take together to find a diagnosis and asked her about her habits and lifestyle.

"First," I said. "We need to confirm this diagnosis."

She looked anxious, asking me, "What do you think this is?"

I sighed. "We'll need to confirm this diagnosis with testing, but my instincts tell me that this is Rheumatoid arthritis."

Georgia's eyes widened, and her chest moved up and down. "Isn't that like—for older people?" she said, and I chuckled.

"Not necessarily—this disease often affects younger people, too," I explained to her. "Once we have the diagnosis, we'll discuss the treatment to help you feel better."

"Is this my fault?" she asked sheepishly.

I took both of her hands in mine with a warm smile on my face. "Of course not, Georgia."

---

1   Please note that all patient names and identifying information have been changed in accordance with California State and federal laws and regulations.

A few weeks later, after Georgia had jumped through a few hoops—bloodwork and an X-ray—my diagnosis was confirmed: She had RA. During her follow-up appointment, we discussed a treatment plan and how we could alleviate her pain, reduce her inflammation, and make her feel better.

What is Rheumatoid Arthritis?

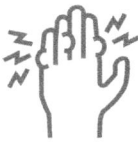

Like Georgia, you might have some questions and misconceptions, especially if your physician is tossing around a scary-sounding diagnosis like Rheumatoid arthritis. Before we discuss the history, treatment, or changes you can make to mitigate RA's impact, let's introduce what RA is on a scientific level.

Rheumatoid arthritis is an autoimmune disease caused by unwelcome changes in your immune system. When functioning normally, your immune system protects your body from invaders like bacteria or viruses. When these invaders, or pathogens, enter your body, your immune system can sense that they're not supposed to be there and attack them. Think of your immune system like a steel shield of armor—its job is to keep you safe from things that might harm you.

Like most shields, your immune system and its cells aren't foolproof.

Sometimes, it makes mistakes, causing autoimmune diseases like RA. Autoimmune diseases occur when your immune system attacks healthy cells. For example, type 1 diabetes, an autoimmune disease, occurs when your immune system attacks the pancreas. In RA, the immune system mistakenly attacks the body's healthy joint tissues, causing inflammation, thickening, and damage. More specifically, immune cells attack the cartilage and bone, leading to swelling, tenderness, and pain. Over time, uncontrolled inflammation can cause irreparable joint destruction and deformity.

Most commonly, RA attacks joints in the hands, wrists, knees, and feet, but may potentially affect all joints. If left untreated, the damage done to the cartilage and bones becomes irreversible and causes chronic pain, deformity, and an inability to use the joints properly.

While joint pain and discomfort are typically among the key reasons bringing patients into my office, RA-related inflammation affects other body systems, including the heart and vessels, the lungs, the eyes, and even the skin.

This widespread inflammation can lead to fatigue, lung and heart diseases, eye problems, and anemia.

Unfortunately, scientists don't yet know the cause of RA or why those who develop it do. That's why, when patients come to me, I assure them that this disease isn't their fault. While some lifestyle components clearly contribute to their symptom severity, it's entirely in their power and in your power to make changes that can help support managing the disease.

Beyond the Prescription Pad: Why Lifestyle Matters

"So—what now?" Georgia asked me with a sigh, a dismayed look crossing her face. Georgia had been coming to me for four months when this conversation happened. After I had diagnosed her with RA, I started her on methotrexate, one of  my go-to clinical treatments for Rheumatoid arthritis (see Chapter 3 for a detailed look at the most common RA treatments available). Unfortunately, it didn't seem to be working—at least, not as effectively as Georgia and I had hoped. When I examined her hands, I noticed unrelenting swelling in her joints. As I mentioned earlier in the book, approximately 60% of RA patients respond to a given treatment plan, and this time, Georgia fell into the unfortunate other 40%.

> ○ **PROTIP**
>
> For best results, treat RA early and aggressively to prevent complications like lung, heart or eyes disease.

I sensed that Georgia would be receptive to my approach to combating the inflammation associated with Rheumatoid arthritis using lifestyle changes. "Well," I began apprehensively. "There are other things we can try, like lifestyle changes."

Georgia's eyes widened. "Really?" she asked. "Do those *really* work?"

I nodded. "Not only does it work, but in some cases, when patients change their diet, exercise plan, and sleep better, they don't need as much medication."

"Where can I find this information?" she asked. "I tried to Google more about it before our appointment, but there is so much information on the Internet. It's impossible to know what's misinformation and what's accurate. Some said that diet changes help, and others said they don't."

I nodded at her again. "That's true—you can't rely on Google." I pulled out a few copies of some research I kept in my drawer. Throughout the rest of her appointment, we discussed the lifestyle changes she could make to help improve her symptoms.

"I've never had a doctor tell me that I can change my diet or workout differently. That's so cool."

Based on our discussions and my advice during the six months that followed, she overhauled her diet, filling it with nutritious foods proven to help fight inflammation. With minimal pharmaceutical treatment, she significantly improved. Georgia's energy levels skyrocketed, her pain disappeared, and she returned to work at her bakery. I was so proud of Georgia's progress, not just because I loved her bakery's cannolis but because true, meaningful change isn't easy. With little intervention on my part, she took a good look at her habits and decided to make choices to benefit herself and her disease. That I couldn't have been more proud of.

This conversation happened early in my career. Today, I would've given Georgia everything lifestyle-related in my toolkit when I first diagnosed her. I didn't know then what I know now: that most patients are more than willing to take matters into their own hands and change their lives for the better.

Let me make one thing clear: I'm not against medical treatment. As a physician with a thriving practice, I prescribe medication every day. But clinical treatments can be a double-edged sword. While they benefit many patients, others find them cumbersome and expensive. That is why, in my practice, I bridge the medications from the traditional, western medicine with my holistic approach that will get my patients to remission faster and with less complications as many of my patients will use just minimal amounts of medications.

Every physician takes the Hippocratic oath the day they become a doctor, and, in my practice, I think of it often. It begins, "By all that I hold highest, I promise my patients competence, integrity, candor, personal commitment to their best interest…" and continues with the sentence, "I shall do by my patients as I would be done by." I wouldn't want the quality of my life intricately tied to expensive pills and trips to the doctor. And, at my core, I don't want my patients to rely on a tiny pill for the rest of their lives. For them, I hope and aim for a fulfilling, enjoyable life free from pain, inflammation, and fatigue. This is the life I seek for myself, and it's the life I prioritize for my patients, whether it's through lifestyle changes alone, or a combination of these changes and medicine.

When you or any patient comes to see me in my office, regardless of your age, occupation, gender, or sexual orientation, you'll hear me speak a great deal about what I know and what science says works for RA. This includes medication, but medication doesn't always solve a patient's problems. My goal is to heal you, and to that end, I'll also discuss nutrition and lifestyle interventions with you.

This surprises most patients, especially if they've seen another rheumatologist before. Many say, "My previous rheumatologist told me that diets don't work for Rheumatoid arthritis," or, "Why has no one told me this before?"

> O **PROTIP**
>
> **If your physician does not mention anything about lifestyle choices, then you should discuss these as complementary to traditional medical treatment.**

Do these statements surprise me? No, not at all! During a physician's training, they spend countless hours recognizing a disease's signs, symptoms, and tests, all to gain a correct diagnosis. Doctors spend a similar amount of time—hundreds if not thousands of hours—learning how to treat patients with the newest, cutting-edge medications. We learn that if one drug doesn't work, we should replace or supplement it with another. But remember what I said earlier in this book: hroughout their ten years (and sometimes more) of training, most rheumatologists spend only a few hours discussing nutrition and exercise, let alone other interventions like mindfulness. We aren't taught about the foods we eat and the impact nutrition has on the body, and I believe this knowledge would help almost all physicians practice better medicine focused on patient *health care*, not patient *sick care*.

The latest American Guidelines on RA only conditionally recommend diet as a part of an RA treatment. Because it isn't strongly recommended, nor do we learn about it, many doctors try to avoid the subject of nutrition altogether. In other words, we disregard it because of a lack of knowledge and understanding. So—if diet isn't reinforced by governing organizations and isn't taught during training, how can we expect physicians to recommend it?

I've gone back to school many times throughout my life, and while I highly value and use my traditional medical training daily, I truly believe in a holistic approach governed by nutrition, mindfulness, exercise, and restful sleep. My goal is to give you all the tools you need to become a better person, patient, friend, and advocate for this disease, and all of those are nestled in the pages of this book.

Google Isn't Your Doctor

RA patients often experience a wide range of physical and emotional symptoms before their first appointment with me, as well as 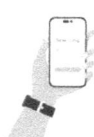 after we begin working together. Many are curious and filled with questions for which they crave fast answers. And some, like Georgia, consult the first thing that pops into their mind—-Google.

Google is sometimes helpful, but it doesn't have years of experience and training as a physician. And, as a whole, the Internet is filled with misinformation–and without the proper training, it's hard to sort our what advice is valuable, what advice is worthless, and most concerningly, what information can be harmful. Unfortunately, when online information is taken as law by desperate patients seeking medical advice, it can become potentially damaging. Too often, I see patients suffer from dire consequences like infections or complications; when I ask them what happened, their first sentence is almost always, "Well, I Googled it, and it said…" In these cases, advice that was ment to help patients was, in truth, harmful to them, and we'll discuss this concept in more depth in Chapter 10.

Try this: Open a browser window and search, "What is the best diet for Rheumatoid arthritis?"

The results are startling and overwhelming. You'll find instructions for vegan diets, paleo diets, keto diets, intermittent fasting, the carnivore diet, and too many others. What's almost worse than misinformation is conflicting information: Each "recommended" diet dismisses the others' value. You'll find many reputable health websites, such as *WebMD, Healthline,* and *Medscape,* but even these offer conflicting information on diets for RA patients.

And, of course, there's social media. On Facebook, Instagram, and TikTok, there is an endless rabbit hole of influencers claiming to be 'autoimmune experts' with different and expensive advice for how to treat RA. The "solution" they're selling you, whether it be an online coaching program, formula, or supplement, can do more harm than good. Though they assure you that what they're telling you is the absolute truth and that their guidance can cure your disease, they aim to make money.

> *Influencers are fantastic salespeople, but they're not doctors.*

These falsehoods aren't anything but garbage. Like all autoimmune diseases, RA is a chronic condition that requires monitoring and adjustments over time. These diseases are complex, often resulting from a combination of factors from inherited genetics, long-term stress on the body's bones and joints, and lifestyle choices. In other words, it takes more than some anecdotal experience or a baseless proclamation to accurately and adequately treat RA.

In contrast, this book results from many years of exploration, trial and error, and thoughtful, caring experiences with my patients. Unlike the "experts" from the internet, I've collected years of training, certifications, and many additional courses in nutrition and mindfulness in addition to my traditional medical training, and my goal is to make this available to you, to help you through the process and ultimately achieve a life free from pain and discomfort.

Just as a structured approach helps us achieve our goals in life, this book offers a structured approach to understanding Rheumatoid arthritis and implementing the changes that lessen inflammation and pain.

Some of the questions I'll answer for you are:

- What causes RA?
- Why am I developing this disease specifically?
- What do I need to change to feel less pain and less inflammation?
- How is the food I eat related to my gut?
- Is RA related to the food I eat?

- Which foods help with my inflammation?
- Are there supplements I can take, and do they work?
- Is stress worsening my pain?
- How can I become less stressed?
- What about exercise—does that help?
- What do I do about my sleep?
- Which remedies *actually* help?
- What does my future look like?

Thus, in 12 chapters, you will have the "what, why, and how" of RA. I'll dispel myths, present the science, and guide you on your Rheumatoid arthritis journey.

I believe in the phrase, "knowledge is power." After all, understanding what's happening motivates us to change and start tackling pain and inflammation problems. So, to tackle these problems, enhance your understanding, and get you started on your symptom-free journey, I've provided you with action steps for each piece of advice. Follow these to improve your health, take less medicine, and feel less pain.

While reading, you will slowly become the CEO of your journey with Rheumatoid arthritis. You can't let Rheumatoid arthritis define how you live and enjoy every day—you have to, and can, take charge. I hope that all the information in this book provides you the support you need to live your best life—free of pain and with renewed understanding.

CHAPTER 2

UNDERSTANDING THE PAST TO IMPROVE THE PRESENT

Diseases like RA have altered the course of history, as has history impacted our modern understanding of RA. Therefore, understanding RA's history is crucial to understand this disease and how it affects you today.

In this section, we'll discuss the history of RA and what causes and exacerbates the condition. We will also cover some common examples of celebrities and athletes fighting this disease just like you.

Then and Now: The History of RA

Dr. Augustin Jacob Landré-Beauvais was the first to write about RA in 1800. While working in a French hospital, Dr. Landré-Beauvais encountered patients with reddened joints and pain in both hands. Other physicians believed that their symptoms were the result of gout, which primarily affected men of high socioeconomic status; however, Landré-Beauvais's patients were women of the same class, which left him confused. Their condition couldn't be explained by other ailments known at the time, and there wasn't yet a name for what these women suffered from. Because of this, Dr. Landré-Beauvais concluded that the condition was uncharacterized and called it "*Goutte Asthénique Primitive*," or "Primary Asthenic Gout." Though he was right to think that this condition was distinct, he was wrong about one thing—RA and gout are entirely different conditions, and we'll discuss this in more detail in the coming chapters.

Later in the 19th century, English doctor Alfred Garrod was the first to distinguish gout from other arthritic conditions affecting his patients; he referred to these other conditions as "rheumatic gout." His son, Archibald Garrod, furthered his father's research and coined "Rheumatoid arthritis" in his 1890 treatise. In his book, *A Treatise On Rheumatism And Rheumatoid Arthritis*, he discusses his findings on ancient skeletons worldwide, including those from ancient Egypt and Greece. The skeletons showed signs of what he called "a new disease," a condition that remained unnamed in medical literature.[1] Unlike skeletons that show signs of gout or other arthritic conditions, the skeletons had symmetrical deformities in their joints, hands, and ankles. His work shows us that RA is nothing new—it's been around for ages.

In the late 1970s, scientists using X-ray technology were finally able to notice differences in the bones of RA patients and those suffering from other arthritic conditions. As Garrod had seen nearly a century prior, bone deformities were symmetrical, affecting both hands or ankles simultaneously. This was a significant breakthrough in medicine, and today, we understand that RA typically affects joints symmetrically.

Much like physicians' understanding of RA as its unique disease, scientific advancements and treatments have come a long way. In the past, RA was treated with bloodletting, cold and hot water therapy, and gold salt therapies, all of which are minimally, if not wholly, ineffective. Treatment has come a long way: New medications are launched every few years, offering patients relief. In the not-so-distant past, RA condemned patients to a life of chronic pain, deformities, and disability. Luckily, because of research efforts and technological improvements, we rarely see the deformities pictured in textbooks in person.

Furthermore, because of relentless research, we understand that medication isn't the only promising solution to RA patient's symptoms. Lifestyle and diet have been proven to be pivotal in how patients manage their condition daily. For example, science has uncovered certain foods that cause flare-ups, such as nightshade vegetables, which we'll discuss in more depth in Chapter 5. More promisingly, research shows that other foods, such as fruit and fiber, can mitigate inflammation and pain.

Lifestyle changes, such as getting more regular exercise, is another important way to help control RA: In the past, commoners worked laborious jobs, and had limited access to transportation. Today, cars and public transport make walking obsolete. We no longer have to walk to work, to the store, or anywhere for that matter, but for those suffering from RA, the lack of exercise that comes with serious side effects. Luckily, science unveils specific exercises, like aquatic therapy, that help fight inflammation and pain.

Because of these advancements, most modern RA patients can control their condition through a combination of clinical treatments, lifestyle changes, and dietary alterations. In the chapters to come, we'll discuss not only the importance of making these healthy changes, but I'll also include actionable tips backed by years of modern scientific research to help you get started.

Famous Faces of RA: Those Who Share the Struggle

Diagnosis and treatment for RA can be tricky—many people don't know where to start. However, many people living today—some of whom you already know—suffer from RA, and they serve as solid examples of the power of proactive treatment, motivation, and the value of lifestyle.

For example, Danielle Collins, a rising star in the tennis world, shocked her fans when, in 2019, she announced that she was diagnosed with Rheumatoid arthritis. Danielle reported that she didn't know what was happening with her body for a while, but that, when she received her diagnosis, she felt relief. Finally, her symptoms were validated!

She told her fans, "As a professional athlete, you are constantly reminded that your body is your temple. My health is of the utmost importance to me, and I'm ready to take on the fight of Rheumatoid arthritis."

So, what did she do? Danielle began incorporating healthier, inflammation-busting foods into her diet and adapted her training schedule to minimize the impact on her joints. Along with her doctors, she worked on her stress levels, continuously adapting to her body's needs to fight her disease. Though she still experiences the occasional flare-up or bout of morning stiffness, today, she lives nearly pain-free and consistently wins on the tennis court.

Another strong example is Terry Bradshaw, the four-time Super Bowl champion and the iconic quarterback for the Steelers team in Pittsburgh, Pennsylvania. When speaking on the condition, Terry warns people that Rheumatoid arthritis has nothing to do with age, saying, "You don't have to be an old athlete like me to wake up with sore joints…as most [autoimmune diseases] don't have anything to do with age".

Over the following years, Terry became a strong advocate for Rheumatoid arthritis. He took a leadership position in the American College of Rheumatology's Simple Tasks campaign to educate others about this disease and regularly speaks out to the millions of people suffering from RA about his experience with the condition.[2]

When speaking on his approach to RA, he speaks with inspiration, saying, "I approach every day, every morning, the same way: jacked up!"

Today, Terry serves as a potent reminder of the value of a positive mindset throughout the RA treatment and diagnosis process.

Unfortunately, not every celebrity struggling with RA has a success story to share. Kathleen Turner, a legendary Hollywood actress known for roles in films like *Peggy Sue Got Married* or *The War of the Roses,* suffers from the condition. For Turner, it began in the 90s with what she called "inexplicable pains and fevers." She found these debilitating, saying, "My body could respond only with excruciating pain whenever I tried to move at all. The joints in my hands were so swollen I couldn't hold a pen. Some days, I couldn't hold a glass to get a drink of water. I couldn't pick up my child… my feet would blow up so badly that I couldn't get them into any kind of shoes, let alone walk on them." Unfortunately, because of the pain, Kathleen couldn't continue her career.

Like many RA patients, Turner struggled to get a diagnosis for her symptoms. And, after a year of inconclusive tests and unanswered questions, she "could hardly turn her head or walk, and was told she would end up in a wheelchair."

Turner's appearance drastically changed after her RA diagnosis, and so did the press she received. She says this of the media at that time, "They snipped that I had become fat and unrecognizable because I was an angry, washed-up diva, an out-of-control has-been, when in truth the changes in my physical appearance were caused by drugs and chemotherapy and were not within my control."

Unlike Bradshaw and Collins, Turner didn't reveal her struggle to the "merciless" public. She allowed the public to assume she was a drinker instead of opening up about her rheumatoid arthritis diagnosis. Of this, she says, "They'd hire me if they thought I was a drunk because they could understand drinking, but they wouldn't hire me if I had a mysterious, scary illness they didn't understand…I felt it was imperative to keep my rheumatoid arthritis quiet."

Unfortunately, her career took a hit for a while, but with the proper treatment, she returned to the screen in the early 2000s. Today, Turner speaks out about her diagnosis. Though she struggled to find a treatment plan that worked for her, she encourages patients to continue trying until something sticks and recommends a personalized approach to their treatment plan.

While these stories are inspiring and relatable, they indicate that anyone, regardless of wealth, health, or age, can develop RA. It doesn't discriminate, and you aren't alone. These famous people battle Rheumatoid arthritis, too, and use their channels to raise awareness about the disease and empower and inspire others. They serve to show that RA diagnosis can be a shock, but with early detection, better understanding, and the development of therapeutic options, you can get better.

Rheumatoid arthritis isn't unbeatable. If they can fight Rheumatoid arthritis, you can as well. Take their hope and pain, and use it to fuel your own journey.

CHAPTER 3

RHEUMATOID ARTHRITIS 101

Many patients feel that Rheumatoid arthritis is a complicated disease shrouded in questions. Physicians and scientists—like myself—understand that it's not genuinely complex; however, to laymen, terms and details can feel confusing and intangible.

Consider this chapter as if you were making a to-do list. All your tasks seem daunting at the beginning of the day: You might have to prepare dinner, deliver a report, get your children ready, etc. But when you break them down while making a to-do list, the steps seem much more manageable. In other words, defrosting tonight's chicken, packing your children's lunches, and blocking out an hour to research your report is much simpler when you decomplicate them.

Some of this information we'll discuss is heavy and maybe a little scary, much like your larger, daunting tasks. However, discussing what, who, why, when, and how makes this abstract information much more tangible. In truth, there's nothing scary about RA, but it and your treatment require a consistent and stepwise approach.

Though we briefly introduced RA in the last chapter, I'm sure you still have many questions, and I aim to answer them. So, in this chapter, we'll cover:

- Who's at risk for RA?
- Common symptoms and causes
- How is RA diagnosed?
- How is RA treated?

In this chapter, we'll decomplicate RA, breaking it down into its smaller, more digestible components to help you understand your disease, and to empower you to make healthy changes to support your healing process.

> *RA, like heart disease, diabetes,*
> *or high blood pressure,*
> *is a condition, not a label.*

Are you ready? Let's get started.

Why Me? Who is Affected By RA?

Rheumatoid arthritis is among the most common autoimmune diseases, affecting about 1% of the global population. Although this number might seem relatively small, there are about 17.6 million people worldwide, 1.4 million of whom reside in the U.S., just like you, working through this disease one step at a time.

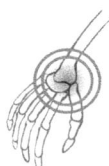

I often receive this question from patients—Why me? My go-to answer is, "Well—why *not* you? RA can happen to anyone!" There's truthfully little rhyme or reason as to why you specifically suffer from RA. You're not just plain ol' unlucky; instead, RA is the result of three things: Genetic predisposition, hormonal mechanisms, and lifestyle.

Instead of boring you with a long list of risk factors, let's discuss Maria, a former patient who checked almost all of the boxes.

When Maria visited my office, she was 45 years old. She, like many patients whom I diagnosed with RA, complained of pain in her hands, accompanied by swelling and persistent morning stiffness. She also noted that she occasionally struck a fever and had hot flashes, and, over the last six months, she'd felt more tired than usual.

Before coming in, Maria filled out a patient questionnaire and a brief family history. When I read her paperwork, I noticed that both Maria's mother and grandmother had suffered from RA. Unfortunately for Maria, genetics play an important role in RA. For example, those with a first-degree relative who suffers from RA (a mother, father, or sibling) like Maria are three times more likely to develop the disease.[1] On the other hand, those with a second-degree relative (grandparent, uncle, or aunt) who suffers from RA are at two times increased risk for developing the disease.

Do you recommend genetic testing for RA?

Answer: NO! Genetic testing is not helping with RA diagnosis and will not influence how patients are treated.

The questionnaire included information about Maria's age and gender, which checked another so-called box in my mind. Women are three times more likely to develop RA compared to men, and this is particularly true for women between the ages of 30 and 60.[2] Scientists aren't sure why this is the case but believe it may be related to the estrogen load and the X chromosome, which contains genes associated with the immune system. Having two X chromosomes increases a person's likelihood of mutations in these genes, making women genetically predisposed to autoimmune disorders.

Maria's age, 45, signaled another potential problem: Scientists have unveiled a link between estrogen, the female sex hormone, and RA.[3] It's theorized that lower estrogen levels raise the body's inflammatory protein levels, causing the condition.[2] So, during menopause, when a woman's estrogen levels dramatically drop, their inflammatory protein levels skyrocket, increasing their risk of developing RA. Contrastingly, during pregnancy when estrogen levels multiply, RA symptoms tend to significantly improve.

Additionally, some studies show that the early onset of menopause (before age 45) is associated with RA.[4] There's also evidence connecting menopause to bone thinning, a cause for concern for arthritis patients. Estrogen helps maintain bone density, and declining estrogen levels can accelerate bone loss. If left untreated, this could lead to other types of arthritis, like osteoarthritis (otherwise referred to as 'wear and tear' arthritis).

Is hormone replacement therapy appropriate as a treatment for RA?

If you have a diagnosis of RA and experience worsening of your symptoms, including menopause signs (hot flashes, mood swings, worsening of the pain, etc), then based on the last guidelines from 2020, the American College of Rheumatology recommends hormone replacement therapy.[5] Be aware that this will complement but will not replace the traditional RA treatment.

I was willing to bet that when Maria had chalked up her early symptoms to menopause. While she wasn't wrong—her hot flashes seemed to indicate menopause—she wasn't entirely correct. Unfortunately, many women make this mistake, believing that their symptoms are menopause and not RA. Some menopause symptoms, like fatigue, night sweats, and hair thinning, the result of hormone changes, are common in both conditions. Furthermore, each condition can cause mood changes, depression, and anxiety. Dry eyes, skin, and mouth are shared between the two, as are sleep issues.

When Maria came into my office, a nurse took her height, weight, and notes about her lifestyle. Maria was just over five feet tall, and weighed over

200 lbs; in other words, her BMI was well over the normal range. Immediately, I understood this to be a problem, not just for her health, but for her potential diagnosis, as research shows that people with a body mass index (BMI) over 30 have a 30% increased risk of developing RA.[6]

Which lifestyle factors are risk factors for RA?
- Smoking
- A poor diet
- Poor dental hygiene
- Lack of physical activity
- Obesity
- Exposure to smoke/second-hand smoking
- Pollution

When asked about her diet, Maria reported that she frequently consumed soda, and ate at home infrequently because of her hectic work schedule. As a result, she relied on fast food and take-out options for most of her meals and beverages. Knowing that overeating sugar, too much salt, or regularly indulging in ultra-processed foods can have a profound effect on who develops RA, I took note of this.[7]

Maria also told the nurse that she was a smoker. Though she'd tried to cut back, she never found herself able to: Her work-related stress was always too much, and Maria would begin smoking just as soon as she'd quit. Smoking is the most decisive lifestyle risk factor for RA,[8] and the habit increases your risk of developing not only RA but also some of its more aggressive forms.[9]

I immediately knew this was an issue, not just at present but in the future. In some cases, smoking can make treatment a little trickier and can potentially decrease your treatment's efficacy—its ability to work. In other words, smokers respond poorly to RA treatment than non-smokers, and I knew that if Maria did have RA, we would need to monitor her treatment closely.

Though Maria never mentioned stress explicitly, she did say her hectic work schedule a few times throughout the conversation. Unfortunately for many of us, stress has been shown to play a role in the development of RA, and is considered a risk factor. Research illustrates that women with posttraumatic stress disorder (PTSD) have an increased risk of developing the disease.[10]

Can COVID-19 virus or vaccine trigger Rheumatoid arthritis?

While some patients have reported developing Rheumatoid arthritis (RA) symptoms after COVID-19 infection or vaccination, the nature of this relationship remains uncertain. Currently, there is no definitive evidence that the COVID-19 virus causes RA. Like other viruses, there might be just an association, not a cause-effect relationship.[11]

What are some other risk factors for RA?

1. **Gut changes:** Differences in gut microbiome (discussed more in Chapter 4) are seen between RA patients and normal individuals. Interestingly, these differences can potentially normalize during RA treatment.

2. **Periodontal disease:** Certain bacterial species, such as Prevotella, are linked to the formation of specific antibodies, like CCP antibodies, that can increase your chances of developing RA.

3. **Vitamin D deficiency:** Data suggests that people deficient in vitamin D are generally at increased risk of developing autoimmune diseases. Broadly speaking, a higher vitamin D intake decreases the risk of developing autoimmune diseases like RA.

4. **Infections:** Viral infections such as EBV (Epstein Barr Virus) and CMV (Cytomegalovirus) were reported in some cases of RA.

All of these were immediate causes for concern. Without having examined her, I understood that, because of Maria's genetic predisposition, hormone changes, and lifestyle habits (high-sugar diet, hectic, high-stress work schedule, and smoking), she likely had RA.

So, while doctors are unsure of what exactly is causing RA, there are some critical risk factors, all of which Maria had, that increase your likelihood of developing this disease. These include a family history, hormone changes, and lifestyle factors. On the other hand, it's also entirely possible to have NONE of these contributing factors and still develop RA: Remember in the last chapter, we introduced Danielle Collins and Terry Bradshaw, both of whom suffer from RA but have none of these. So it's entirely possible to have no family history of RA, eat a plant-based diet, never touch a cigarette, and still develop the disease.

Who develops RA depends on various factors, which means we have a variety of levers to pull to help control the disease. In other words, if you have a strong family history of the disease, don't fear. While you can't change your genes, you can change how you live your life. Many risk factors, including diet, smoking, and stress, are entirely in your control, and we'll discuss these in detail in the chapters to come.

RA Day-to-Day: What to Expect

After "Why me?" patients usually ask me, "What should I expect?" Everyone is different, but in most cases, patients begin seeing signs of RA in their hands or feet. Most experience the gradual onset of symptoms over a few weeks or months. Their joints can become swollen, red, and warm to the touch.

In 90% of cases, RA attacks a patient's small joints (their hands and feet). Sometimes, it impacts larger joints, like their wrists, shoulders, knees, and ankles. Elbows and hips are affected in about 40% of patients. These larger joints are rarely the first ones affected, and this is usually only in cases in which a patient's disease is more prolonged.

Symmetrical and bilaterally affected joints are most commonly a sign of RA, just like early physicians noticed in the 19th and 20th centuries. In layman's terms, the same joints in a patient's hands or feet are affected simultaneously or on both sides of the body.

So—how does this affect your day-to-day life? Most often, patients start to experience difficulty with daily activities. Sometimes, they struggle to hold their morning coffee, can't type well on a keyboard, or find making a fist difficult. If a patient's feet are affected, they might have difficulty getting out of bed or walking. An inability to move correctly or 'as usual' and pain are among the key reasons patients go to my office.

Sometimes, these symptoms appear seemingly overnight—the patient wakes up one morning stiff as a rock, and can't move their hands like they could just the previous day. Other patients find symptoms onset gradually until they can no longer deny them. Less commonly, RA manifests as swelling and pain in just one joint, such as the wrist or the knee, and then jumping to the other wrist/ knee, shoulders, knees, ankles, and feet. Because this type of arthritis moves from one place to another, we call this *"migratory" arthritis.*

Figure 1. Areas affected by RA (bilateral and symmetric involvement of the joints including the small joints in the hands, wrists, feet but also big joints like shoulders, elbows,

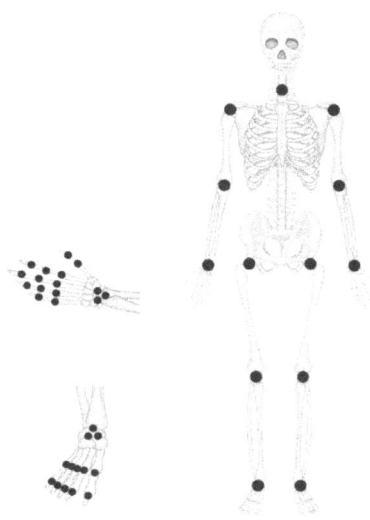

Figure 1. Areas affected by RA (bilateral and symmetric involvement of the joints including the small joints in the hands, wrists, feet but also big joints like shoulders, elbows, knees and ankles)

RA can occur in flare-ups too: In some patients, symptoms come on like an attack, lasting just a few days or weeks. Attacks, or flare-ups, usually resolve on their own or with an over-the-counter anti-inflammatory medication. At first, patients find flare-ups more intermittent, but over time, frequency increases, and these attacks can become more debilitating.

Which Symptoms Should I Expect?

Beyond the characterizing joint inflammation and pain, morning stiffness is another sign of inflammation. Often, morning stiffness is long-lived, lasting more than an hour. As the day progresses, moving your hands, stretching your muscles, or walking will decrease some stiffness in the hands and feet. The pain may persist in the joints, but you'll feel less stiff.

While pain and swelling in the joints are the most frequent complaints bringing patients into my office, I occasionally see patients who develop fevers, lose significant amounts of weight, and report feeling very weak and severely fatigued. These, too, along with pain and redness, are signs of inflammation taking over the whole body.

What About the UNCOMMON Signs and Symptoms of RA?

Check out the boxes for some of these signs, and how they unfold.

Low-grade fevers Persistent low-grade fevers might be your body's means of reacting to inflammation. However, fevers can be a sign of infection or a side effect from a certain medication.	**Overwhelming fatigue** Many patients report a fatigue that negatively impacts their daily life, work performance, and sex drive. Often a sign of uncontrolled inflammation, fatigue can be a consequence of insomnia and depression.
Gum disease Individuals with poor oral hygiene are more likely to develop RA. And, if a patient's RA isn't well-managed, they can develop gum disease.	**Neck pain** RA can affect the neck, causing pain, stiffness, and difficulty moving the head. Pain that radiates down from the neck to the arms needs further evaluation as this can be a severe complication of RA.
Bilateral carpal tunnel syndrome In most cases, patients experience carpal tunnel syndrome on their dominant hand. Don't jump into surgical options just yet—in my practice, I've seen many patients who have undergone surgery on both hands when RA is truly to blame.	**Jaw pain or temporomandibular joint (TMJ) pain** Also referred to as TMJ, this symptom is seen in about 30-50% of RA patients. TMJ can cause facial and ear pain, headaches, difficulties in opening the mouth fully, and clicking noises that accompany jaw movement.
Dry eyes and mouth These symptoms are referred to as secondary Sjögren's Syndrome, and are common when inflammation is poorly controlled. Patients report a "gritty, sand-like sensation" in their eyes and increased thirst due to severe dry mouth.	**Raynaud's disease** Raynaud's causes a change in the color of your fingers or toes, and sometimes affects nose or ears. Fingers turn bluish as the blood supply in these areas decreases and then reddens again with blood flow.
Voice changes Hoarseness or other voice changes can be seen in about 30% of patients, occuring when when inflammation affects the larynx (or the *cricoarytenoid joint*).	**Other uncommon symptoms** Depression and anxiety Muscle weakness Eye inflammation Skin rashes

As I previously mentioned, pain is the common denominator in bringing patients into my office, but it certainly isn't the only motivator. So—what about uncommon signs and symptoms?

Beyond pain and redness, sometimes, patients show signs of inflammation, and they don't even know it. When I interview patients, I identify other signs that point towards inflammation, such as dryness in their eyes or mouth, severe fatigue, carpal tunnel syndrome, vocal changes, gum disease, or depression. All of these are signs of inflammation's effect on your other body systems.

How Is RA Diagnosed?

Too commonly, patients battle pain, swelling, and stiffness for months or even years before reaching a specialist's office. Many believe that their pain will go away; they take some over-the-counter painkillers or antiinflammatories, and soon, the pain subsides. But these medications do not address the problem—just mask it. Other people blame their age, their job, or the stress they put on their bodies and put off seeking help.

When the pain doesn't go away, most patients first seek the help of their Primary Care Physician (PCP). Usually, their doctor orders an initial set of blood tests and X-rays before referring them to a rheumatologist. So, months pass before patients are seen by the specialist who can diagnose them.

In the case of RA, as in medicine, a bird's eye view of the patient's struggle yields more valuable results than a simple blood test.

RA is a clinical diagnosis, meaning that only a trained doctor can adequately assess the patient's symptoms and medical history (risk factors), and run tests to conclude that the patient suffers from RA.

A doctor must follow these steps and employ a zoomed-out perspective of the patient to make sure to get critical evidence, leading to misdiagnosis. For example, specific blood tests, such as Rheumatoid factor tests, can come back positive, and even so, positive blood tests without clinical symptoms don't necessarily mean Rheumatoid arthritis (RA). Laboratory and imaging tests are imperfect and don't always provide a clear image of the patient's struggles. Sometimes, symptoms are general and indicative of any ailments, with RA being only one. So, misdiagnosis is relatively common, particularly if the doctor doesn't follow the proper steps.

> ○ **PROTIP**
>
> It's important to know that positive tests without clinical signs and symptoms do not mean that you have a disease. The reverse is also true: Signs and symptoms that are suggestive of RA, while blood tests are negative, does not exclude the diagnosis.

The Journey to Diagnosis

Diagnosis follows a relatively straightforward path, beginning with blood tests, followed by more in-depth imaging studies, including X-rays and, if needed, MRIs, to glean a more robust understanding of the problem at hand and the severity of the patient's RA.

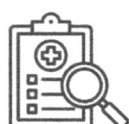

First, your doctor will likely run a blood panel, and the results can point to any number of physical conditions. For example, a blood test can indicate infections, anemia, leukemia, or dehydration.

Because they yield such broad results, physicians have to zoom in—as though with a metaphorical microscope—and look at the results of more specific tests run in the whole panel. More specific tests include inflammation markers, Rheumatoid factor (RF), anti-CCP antibodies (CCP stands for cyclic citrullinated peptide), and Antinuclear antibodies (ANA) tests.

Common laboratory tests for RA
• Cell Blood Counts
• Liver panel
• Kidney panel
• Rheumatoid factor (RF)
• Anti-CCP antibodies
• Antinuclear Antibodies (ANA)
• Erythrocyte Sedimentation Rate (ESR)
• C-reactive protein (CRP)
• Hepatitis Panel, Parvovirus

Inflammation marker tests are ordered to evaluate the patient for inflammation. Typical inflammation markers include Erythrocyte Sedimentation Rate (ESR) and C-reactive protein (CRP). Elevated levels usually indicate that a patient is currently experiencing joint pain or swelling.

The Rheumatoid Factor (commonly abbreviated as RF) test can be a little tricky: While this test is positive in about 60-70% of patients with RA, this leaves between 30-40% of patients with a negative result. It's important to note that you may still suffer from RA despite a negative test result. Furthermore, it's essential to understand that a positive RF test can be seen in conditions like Sjogren's Disease, Infections (Hepatitis B or C), Lymphomas, or even in ordinary people.

> **What is Rheumatoid arthritis with a negative rheumatoid factor test?**
>
> About 50% of patients with RA have Rheumatoid factor and anti-CCP antibodies negative tests at the time of their disease's onset.
>
> We call this "Seronegative" Rheumatoid arthritis; over time, some of these cases are identified as other forms of arthritis, such as psoriatic arthritis or ankylosing spondylitis.
>
> However, about 20% of patients with RA remain without a positive test, and the diagnosis is based on the clinical signs only.

The anti-CCP antibodies (stands for cyclic citrullinated peptide antibodies) test is often ordered along with Rheumatoid Factor. This test has a high specificity, which is doctor-speak because, if a patient's anti-CCP antibody test is negative, their likelihood of having RA is slim.

When both RF and anti-CCP antibodies are positive, patients are most likely diagnosed with RA.

These are by no means the only tests involved. Doctors must rule out other conditions that can mimic inflammatory arthritis, like parvovirus, hepatitis B, C, tuberculosis, Lyme, and HIV, all of which can mimic RA, and cause a positive RF test.

Any other necessary tests?

In the medical community, there is an ongoing debate about whether we should or not order an ANA (antinuclear antibodies) test. In my experience, an ANA test is critical, as its results can rule out other autoimmune diseases (e.g., lupus or Sjogren's). An ANA test can also help me adjust a patient's therapy. For example, if the ANA test is positive, I avoid specific treatments like TNF-alpha inhibitors that may cause further side effects in these patients.

Adding points to make the RA diagnosis

- Rheumatologists, including myself, use specific criteria to make an RA diagnosis. Check out the following criteria for RA diagnosis (I'll link our 2010 guidelines for those eager to learn more):
- Count the number of small or large joints showing signs of inflammation (the more you have involved, the higher the score in points we'll assign). You'll be given a score between 1 and 5.
- Look for elevated markers of inflammation (0-1 points), positive Rheumatoid factor, or anti-CCP antibodies (if they are present, we will assign more points). 1-3 points are assigned based on these criteria.
- Lastly, if the patient has been experiencing them for more than six weeks, we assign another point.
- When doctors put all these pieces together, we can put together the diagnosis. A total of 6/10 points is needed for an RA diagnosis.

What Are the Most Common Imaging Tests for RA?

Imaging comes just after blood tests. Most physicians will use X-rays, Ultrasound, and, in some cases, MRI (magnetic resonance imaging) to understand what's happening inside the body, and to use it as a potential comparative measure.

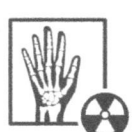

X-rays are my go-to test; when a patient comes to my office, I recommend an X-ray to see if the patient has some bone damage (called erosions) and to establish a disease baseline, which allows me to compare the state of your disease today to what it might be in the future. Let's say two years ago, your X-rays didn't show any erosions. However, when I repeated the X-ray yesterday, erosions riddle your joints. In other words, X-rays show me what blood tests can't—they indicate whether or not a patient's treatment is effective or if we need to alter the dosage or change the medication entirely.

Physicians may also use ultrasound imaging if the X-rays don't show any changes but the patient has persistent symptoms. Ultrasounds are non-invasive methods that capture tendons, ligaments, muscles, and bones using high-frequency sound waves.

When you undergo an ultrasound, the doctor will apply a gel on top of your joint and use a probe to look at the structures below the skin. This practice helps to detect inflammation (called synovitis), crystals (which can distinguish RA from gout), tendon ruptures, or bone erosions.

Despite the real-time nature of the ultrasound and the lack of radiation involved in the study, few U.S. rheumatologists use musculoskeletal ultrasound for diagnostic purposes. This method is used more commonly in Europe.

MRI is reserved for complicated situations, like Thomas, a 61-year-old patient of mine. Thomas battled bilateral joint pain and minor swelling in his large and small knuckles. He struggled to brush his teeth in the mornings, couldn't hold his cup of coffee, or button his own shirt because of the pain. Thomas found his feet bothersome, and he had difficulties going to the restroom.

Before seeing me, he'd seen another rheumatologist who diagnosed him with Osteoarthritis—otherwise known as 'wear and tear' arthritis. Unfortunately, Thomas insisted that his pain and stiffness were worsening but seemed to improve throughout the day generally. Nevertheless, he was in daily, unrelenting pain.

When I examined him, I wasn't too impressed by my own clinical findings: Deformities in his hands could've been related to wear and tear arthritis. In other words, nothing was pointing me to RA.

Thomas insisted that he'd experienced episodes like this one, and, most of the time, they subsided within a few weeks. However, this time, his symptoms had persisted for nearly six months.

Before he arrived at my office, his PCP ordered blood tests: His Rheumatoid factor, anti-CCP antibodies, and markers of inflammation were all normal. X-rays of his hands showed just a few wear and tear changes—not causes for concern. I knew that something wasn't right, so I decided to get an MRI of his right hand.

Sure enough, my gut was right: Thomas has clear signs of inflammation in his small joints in the hands and wrist. He had Rheumatoid arthritis despite multiple negative tests.

Thomas's case represents the importance of using multiple diagnostic tools to assemble the puzzle pieces. While his signs weren't so clear, and while the blood tests were dismissive, the MRI revealed his true diagnosis.

The Dangers of Google

Before they come for a consultation, many of my patients have already Googled the symptoms they're experiencing and, sometimes, the laboratory tests. Because of this, they have pre-formulated ideas about what they might have. Unfortunately, as was the case for Alysa, a 64-year-old patient of mine, they're also left scared and confused by the misleading information they find online.

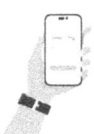

I heard Alysa's story when she came to me after a long, arduous battle with pain. She had a long history of both anxiety and depression, both of which can be risk factors for RA, but when this story unfolded, she was being treated by a therapist and seemed to be doing relatively well. However, she'd begun experiencing joint pain in her elbows, which progressed to her wrists; after a few weeks, she felt pain in her knuckles or the small and large joints in her hands.

When the pain became unbearable, Alysa called her PCP, who scheduled her for an appointment in three weeks. Those three weeks couldn't come soon enough for Alysa; she waited, in severe pain, and began looking up her symptoms on the internet and found something called tendonitis. Throughout those few weeks, Alysa started taking over-the-counter medications—Tylenol and Ibuprofen—to cope with her pain. She Googled her symptoms and found an ad recommending a 'natural' willow bark supplement. She took this daily, thinking nothing of it or her over-the-counter medication use.

Finally, her appointment came. Her doctor, along with regular blood tests, ordered some additional ones to check out her liver and kidney function, and thank goodness he did: Because of her medication use, her kidneys and liver were suffering. Her liver enzymes were elevated, a sign of inflammation or damage, and her kidney function had become affected by the medications she was taking. When Alysa came to me, she was struggling with both of these issues, and I delivered to her the news that she had RA.

When she told me this story, I was overwhelmed with empathy: I understand that patients have questions and that they need to cope with the pain they're experiencing. Alysa hadn't known or understood the risks of these medications and believed they were fine just because she didn't need a prescription to purchase them. Like many others, she was wrong, and I wished I could've done something to help.

The earlier chapters discussed the potential dangers of Googling your symptoms. While looking up your symptoms online isn't necessarily bad and can yield important information, I suggest that anything you learn online should be used as a foundation for discussion with your physician–not as a way to self-diagnosis. Self-diagnosis without consulting with a physician who has the training to assess your symptoms, and who will order the appropriate tests, and knowledge about how even over-the-counter drugs and supplements can impact your body, can leave patients in a similar position to Alysa, with more problems than she'd had to begin with.

Curiosity is merely part of the human condition, and some patients simply can't wait until their appointment for the information they crave. But comments on internet forums and ads couched as suggestions only harm patients, leaving them in a worse position with more damage than they were in previously. I cannot emphasize enough: Googling your symptoms is seemingly innocuous, but can be hazardous without a doctor's oversight.

In the next section, we'll discuss the importance of treatment and the various medications available to you. Hopefully, you will find a little hope in knowing that the pain you're feeling can and will—with a bit of work with your doctor and some lifestyle changes—come to an end.

How Is RA Treated? The Old, New, and Future

Let's say you finally have the RA diagnosis. What's next? Most patients feel relieved when they finally know what's causing their symptoms, but confusion will follow.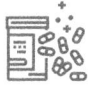

For patients, starting treatment is a difficult feat. Some feel more open and determined to change aspects of their lifestyle to help themselves and their disease, but others are afraid of trying any medication; they take the negative experiences of others and allow that to influence their decision. Some blame doctors and their relationship with pharmaceutical companies, saying they'll profit off of their suffering, while others are ready to swallow the magic pill to relieve the pain. In my experience, neither of these opposite reactions is optimal.

Treatment can be a scary process, especially without the proper information. Worrying about it just raises your blood pressure and your anxiety level! Without a diagnosis, trying proper treatments is like shooting an arrow into the dark and trying to get the target.

Will you hit it?

Most likely—no!

The RA treatment success rate is about 60%, so it's essential to understand that treatment won't cure your disease but instead slows its progression and prevents inflammation from damaging your organs. This book is not anti-medication but rather a bridge between medications used for RA and lifestyle options. There are many ways to manage your RA symptoms, and not all of them are pills or expensive drugs. Diet and lifestyle changes can alter and impact your RA and its symptoms for the better. As I often say, you are the CEO of your RA, and even when hope is lost, you can still make changes to get better.

Living Without Treatment: What Can Go Wrong?

In short, a lot can go wrong if you aren't properly diagnosed and don't receive the right treatment, including with drugs that are clinically proven to control the progression of RA. Before we discuss common treatments, let's talk about the importance of drug therapy in the first place.

Picture inflammation like a giant, looming, uncontrollable fire. If left untamed, the fire is sure to cause severe foreseeable consequences. If we're talking about a house fire, the fire will destroy a wall (or a joint, in this metaphor), then the four walls of an entire room (multiple joints). Over time, if it isn't extinguished, the fire will spread to the house's other rooms; inflammation will affect your lungs, heart, and eyes. Eventually, it will burn down the whole house, leaving only ash in its wake.

Take Evelyn's story for example: Evelyn, an 82-year-old woman who had been dealing with Rheumatoid arthritis (RA) for about 35 years, came to the hospital due to pain and severe changes in her vision, affecting her right eye more than her left. At the hospital, Evelyn showed significant deformities in her hands and feet as a result of RA, and she reported that the only treatment she was using was massive doses of aspirin—only used when she couldn't withstand the pain.

I examined Evelyn's eyes and noticed that she had very thin sclerae (this is the white part of the eyes), and I urgently consulted an eye specialist. Unfortunately, the ophthalmologist confirmed my suspicion— Evelyn had developed a severe eye condition called scleromalacia due to ongoing inflammation linked to RA. She was now in danger of losing her vision and needed immediate surgical intervention.

Evelyn, like a lot of my patients, have a high pain tolerance, and found herself living day-to-day trying to control the pain of a disease she didn't fully understand. Her case is just one example of what I often, and unfortunately, see: Untreated RA can have multiple, very severe consequences. Let's discuss the most common complications of uncontrolled inflammation. It's heartbreaking that Evelyn lived for so long without medication that could have not only stopped the progression of her disease before it impacted her eyes, but also helped spare her pain and deformation of her hands.

Eye problems are common in patients with RA, and if you develop redness, pain, or visual changes, seek urgent evaluation by an eye specialist. These symptoms could be a sign of Scleritis (inflammation of the sclerae, the white part of your eyes). In some cases, the inflammation can cause worse problems, like thinning of the sclerae (called scleromalacia), a severe complication.

Patients with RA often develop dry eyes and mouth, a secondary form of Sjogren's Disease. A dry mouth can also lead to gum disease due to a lack of saliva.

Bone thinning, referred to as osteopenia, can develop in RA patients. However, in time, this condition can become very severe and can cause osteoporosis, which places you at increased risk of developing fractures.

Many patients experience muscle weakness, which could be the effect of disease-causing inflammation in the joints or a side effect from the medications patients use to treat the inflammation.

Can medication cause weakness?

Yes, medications like hydroxychloroquine (Plaquenil), steroids (used in high doses for a long time), or cholesterol-lowering medication (statins) may cause muscle weakness.

Some patients develop heart complications due to ongoing inflammation related to untreated RA. In some cases, inflammation can cause premature atherosclerosis and an increased risk of heart disease.[12] Each of these, unfortunately, can cause early heart attacks and even heart failure. Furthermore, some emergency medications, like NSAIDs and steroids, leave a patient with a higher risk of these conditions. Luckily, methotrexate and TNF inhibitors can lower your risk.

RA untreated—what's the risk?
- Heart and lung disease
- Eye problems
- Thinning of the bones
- Muscle weakness
- Joint deformities
- Chronic pain
- Nodules

Patients with RA can potentially develop lung complications from the disease itself or the use of medications. Methotrexate, Leflunomide, and TNF alpha inhibitors, all of which we'll discuss in the next section, can potentially cause lung disease, though only in rare situations. Your doctor will monitor you for this, again, balancing the effects of RA itself against rare side effects of medications.

Skin conditions are relatively uncommon but can cause anything from RA patients pinpoint rashes to skin ulcerations and vasculitis (inflammation in the small vessels of the skin). Some patients develop some nodules under the skin called rheumatoid nodules. Rheumatoid nodules are a sign of more aggressive disease. Still, sometimes, they may be a side effect of methotrexate medication. It can be confusing that symptoms of the disease itself and the side-effects of the medications to treat it can overlap! You doctor will play an objective role for you, helping to weigh the benefits and risks of treatment.

What are some rare RA complications?
- Kidney issues
- Depression
- Headaches
- Severe anemia
- Low white blood cells
- Low platelets
- Lymphoma (a type of blood cancer)

As I previously mentioned, pain is the critical symptom most often bringing patients into my office. Sometimes, if a patient's pain tolerance is high, they decide to postpone the treatment (remember Evelyn's case), delaying the appropriate window of opportunity to slow down and stop the disease from progressing. By that time, the damage done to their joints is irreversible.

> ## ○ PROTIP
> You can avoid many complications of RA if you start treatment and lifestyle changes early and aggressively.

Often, when patients with long-term or untreated RA come to my office, I'm placed in a position in which I have to share with them bad news about their disease's progression. And, oftentimes, even this isn't enough to convince them to seek treatment. When RA progresses, the deformities that have already developed can't be reversed. So, it's critical for patients and providers not to focus on how the hands or feet look, focusing instead on the loss of proper function. Difficulty using hands to eat, dress, wash, and struggle with daily routine activities is a sign of grave concern.

I'd like you to remember this: Every organ that suffers from ongoing inflammation leaves you at risk for more damage. This is such a pity, as we have great solutions that can help—taking action early and finding a treatment plan that works for you. In some patients, wisely used medications will be your ally—your fire extinguisher—to calm the 'fire' and stop more damage. A fire extinguisher isn't all you need either, and it won't keep the fire from returning. Some solutions don't come in pill form, but rather in changes, you can make entirely on your own. In other words, your lifestyle choices are essential to keep the fire away.

Current Treatments: What's Out There?

Unlike patients in the past, today, you can access treatments that are not only effective, but are scientifically proven to stop the progression of RA. You no longer have to suffer from the ailments and deformities you see in textbooks or online.

In this section, I will briefly discuss current treatments for RA and explain their individual benefits and risks. Remember that this isn't an exhaustive list, and there are various lifestyle changes and shifts you can make to supplement, decrease the need for aggressive medications, decrease the dosage, or lower your use of multiple medications. Check out the later chapters of this book for more information, but for now, feel free to browse this list for a bit of guidance.

DISCLAIMER: This content will briefly cover medications commonly used to treat RA. While we will touch upon the risks and benefits of these medications, please be aware that the information provided needs to be more comprehensive. Understanding that this content is optional for professional medical consultation is essential. You should always consult your physician to discuss medication choices, dosages, and potential side effects, as they may vary significantly based on your individual's specific medical history.

NSAIDS (Non-steroidal anti-inflammatories)

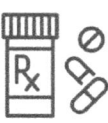

Aspirin, ibuprofen, naproxen, meloxicam, celecoxib, and diclofenac are some of the most common medications RA patients use to alleviate their pain. Some of these are readily available over the counter, but others, like celecoxib, require a medical prescription.

Most of the time, these painkillers take the pain's edge off, and temporarily reduce inflammation. But these medications are not formulated to stop the disease's progression.

Benefits: Pain control, relatively quick effect to decrease pain, easily accessible to patients and family physicians.

Risks: If used for an extended period, these medications can increase the risk of gastric ulcers, gastrointestinal bleeding, kidney failure, liver damage, heart attacks, stroke, and even heart failure. Over-the-counter medications can be especially dangerous because many patients do not fully understand that status as "over-the-counter" does not mean they are without risk.

Steroids

Prednisone, prednisolone, kenalog, and methylprednisolone are today's most potent anti-inflammatory medications. They're fast-acting and relieve pain, swelling, and stiffness in a matter of days. Patients think I am an angel when I give them steroids because, in just a short period of time, they regain access to their lives.

However, we can't treat RA with steroids long-term. As tremendous and positive as their short-term effect can be, using them in high doses long-term is very dangerous. Steroids can be used in combination with other medications or when patients have an RA flare-up, but my advice is to use steroids wisely.

Benefits: They have a powerful anti-inflammatory effect, quickly decreasing inflammation, pain, and swelling, and, in some small doses, might have an immunomodulatory effect (meaning they can decrease the effect of an active immune response in attacking your body).

Risks: They can cause weight gain, diabetes, bone thinning, an increase in blood pressure, gastric ulceration, bleeding, acne, swelling of the legs, easy bruising, increased risk of infections, bone fractures, glaucoma, cataracts, muscle weakness, psychosis, anxiety, and depression (to name a few).

> **What should I know about medication?**
>
> The stronger the medication, the higher its risks. And, the newer the medication is, the less doctors know about its long-term side effects. Patients see medications, including biologics, advertised on TV, but the running, happy people in the ad are not always the reality.
>
> Some of these drugs can increase your risk of developing severe infections, and others just might not be appropriate for your case.
>
> The cost of these medications can be another limiting factor: Some medications cost up to $100,000 a year, and healthcare insurance doesn't approve of a medication until trying another.
>
> Trust your doctor, discuss your options, and keep an open mind.

DMARDs

DMARD stands for disease-modifying antirheumatic drugs. This is a long name, but if you look at its meaning, you'll realize these drugs influence (and stop) the progression of RA. Four drugs are included in this category: methotrexate, leflunomide, hydroxychloroquine, and sulfasalazine. Let's look at each briefly:

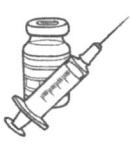

1. **Methotrexate:** This is one of the oldest drugs used in rheumatology; it's about 50 years old now. When patients hear methotrexate, most become alert as they recognize this name as the "cancer drug." However, like aspirin for preventing heart attacks (in a small dose under 81 mg), we also use aspirin to decrease inflammation in higher doses (325-500 mg). For patients with RA, in the case of methotrexate, we use much lower doses (up to 20 mg/ week) compared to the amount used for patients with a cancer diagnosis. So, don't be scared! Talk to your rheumatologist to determine if methotrexate is a good option for you.

   Methotrexate may be given as a pill or injection weekly. It is always best to take it with folic acid, which has been proven to alleviate potential side effects.

   Benefits: Modulates the immune system to decrease inflammation. About 60% of patients who receive only methotrexate respond to this treatment. With very close monitoring, this drug is safe and efficient.

   Risks: The most common side effects of methotrexate are nausea, vomiting, diarrhea, fatigue, bruising, anemia, decreased white blood cells, and liver or kidney damage. It should be avoided entirely if planning a pregnancy or during pregnancy. Two methods of contraception are best to use for women during their childbearing age to prevent this medication's potential effect on your baby in the case of an unplanned pregnancy.

How often should I do blood tests?

While on therapy with most DMARDs (methotrexate, leflunomide, sulfasalazine), you should carefully monitor your blood tests every month for about three months after you start therapy and then continue with them every three months.

2. **Leflunomide:** This is very similar in action to methotrexate. I often call it "methotrexate's sister." This daily pill has very similar benefits and risks to methotrexate. Please refer to the risks and benefits of using methotrexate.

3. **Hydroxychloroquine**: This drug was famous after the COVID-19 pandemic because its role and benefits were debated for COVID-19 patients. Hydroxychloroquine can be given alone in cases of mild arthritis or combined with methotrexate, leflunomide, and even sulfasalazine. The effect is slow: It may take up to 4-6 weeks to see its impact, and it's available in pill form.

   Benefits: Hydroxychloroquine rarely negatively impacts the immune system, and lowers the risk of infections. However, it's slow-acting.

   Risks: Abdominal pain, cramping, diarrhea, hemolytic anemia (some genetically predisposed patients), muscle weakness, skin/ hair discoloration, rash, and headaches. Visual changes and the risk of developing changes related to your eyes are usually dose-dependent and time-dependent. The higher the dose and the longer you are on this medication, the higher the risk of developing eye complications. Rheumatologists know of these possible complications, and we adjust the drug dose based on the patient's weight. We also recommend yearly eye exams and stopping/avoiding therapy in cases of concern. The risk of retinopathy is about 4% after 10 years of use and 8% after 20 years of use.[13]

4. **Sulfasalazine:** This medication is indicated in patients who do not tolerate or have a contraindication for methotrexate or leflunomide. It can also be used to replace hydroxychloroquine.

○ **PROTIP**

DMARDs are drugs that can be used as single therapy, or they can be combined as triple therapy (methotrexate+/-leflunomide+hydroxychloroquine + sulfasalazine) or be combined with biologics.

Biologics

As they became more knowledgeable about the molecules causing inflammation in our body, researchers designed more sophisticated and targeted therapies. Many of these molecules are called "monoclonal antibodies," which are synthetic or humanized proteins designed to counteract (like antibodies) other proteins responsible for creating inflammation (e.g., TNF-alpha and IL-6 proteins). The biologics below are infusions (administered as intravenous therapies) or self-injectables (subcutaneous, prefilled syringes to be administered at home).

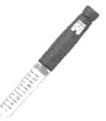

Based on the type of protein they inhabit they are classified as

1. **TNF alpha inhibitors** (e.g., Adalimumab/ Humira, Etanercept/Enbrel, Golimumab/Simponi, Certolizumab/ Cimzia, Infliximab/ Remicade, etc.). These drugs can be used either alone or in combination with methotrexate. The combination is considered superior to using either of these medications alone.
2. **IL-6 inhibitors** (e.g., Tocilizumab/ Actemra and Sarilumab/ Kevzara)
3. **CTLA-4 inhibitors** (Abatacept/ Orencia) inhibit specific immune system cells (T-cells) from interacting with one another and causing more inflammation.

> **Notes on biologics**
> - If you develop an infection during biologic therapy, contact your doctor. Stop your treatment while being treated for the infection, and resume once it's cleared. Keep your doctor 'in the loop' throughout the process.
> - Biologics can be safely combined with other medications, such as methotrexate/leflunomide. Don't stop taking your other medications unless you've been instructed to do so by your physician.
> - If you have a history of cancer, heart disease, or heart failure, tell your doctor. This impacts which therapy is chosen for you.
> - If you're planning a pregnancy, discuss this with your doctor. Certain biologics, like TNF-alpha inhibitors, are considered relatively safe for pregnancy. However, I highly recommend contacting your physician if you plan to conceive or become pregnant.

While the effects and benefits of biologics seem promising, I also tell patients to proceed with caution—these medications can be highly expensive (tens of thousands of dollars a year). These medications also require specific laboratory tests before usage to avoid reactivation of Hepatitis B and C and tuberculosis. For example, patients with evidence of Hepatitis B require frequent monitoring of their viral loads while treated with these drugs. In patients with Hepatitis C, treating the disease before starting a biologic medication is preferred.

Furthermore, vaccinations are recommended before starting biologics therapy: Since these medications can potentially decrease your ability to fight infections, you should get up to date on vaccines to protect you from flu, COVID-19 infection, shingles, or pneumonia. Certain drugs, like JAK inhibitors (see next section), may increase your risk of developing shingles, so it is best to get the shingles vaccine dose before starting these.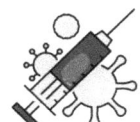

> ○ **PROTIP**
>
> It is recommended that you get up-to-date on vaccines (e.g. pneumonia, COVID-19, flu and shingles vaccine) before starting therapy with DMARDs or biologics.

DMARDs and biologics need time to work—don't expect to feel better overnight! Usually, it takes four to six months to see the effects of these drugs. However, many patients feel better gradually and notice improvement in pain, stiffness, and swelling in a few months.

Benefits: Targeted therapy towards specific molecules that create inflammation. They can act quickly and relieve symptoms, and many patients achieve remission quicker with their use.[14] However, only about 60% of patients benefit from these drugs. In most cases, they are well tolerated but can lose efficacy with long-term use.

What is considered *remission* in RA?

If you have one or fewer tender or swollen joints, if markers of inflammation are normal, you feel as good as usual, and your physician does not find signs of active disease, you are likely in remission.

Risks: Injection site reactions, increased risk of infections (most of the time upper respiratory infections, otitis, sinusitis, and skin infections, more rare severe infections), increases the risk of tuberculosis or hepatitis B/ C, herpes virus reactivation, skin cancer (my recommendation is to have an annual skin exam while on these drugs) are all concerns with these medications. Rarely do they cause an increased risk of lymphoma or other cancers (this is an ongoing debate since ongoing inflammation and carrying an autoimmune disease will also increase the risk of cancer).

Small molecules drugs

Janus kinase (JAK) inhibitors are small, orally-administered active drugs 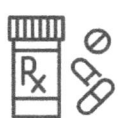 called *targeted synthetic disease-modifying antirheumatic drugs* (tsDMARDs). Sounds fancy, right? They act on the nucleus of immune cells to inhibit the production of multiple proteins that cause inflammation (these are called **cytokines**).

Unlike biologics, which inhibit one molecule at a time (e.g., TNF alpha or IL-6), JAK inhibitors inhibit multiple cytokines at the same time (e.g., IL-6, IL-11, IL-20, interferon-gamma, etc.). These drugs are pills, not injectables.

Benefits: These drugs are convenient, and involve the use of just one pill a day. They work quickly and yield a positive effect on about 60% of RA patients. Our current rheumatology guidelines recommends the use of JAK inhibitors typically after people fail therapy with DMARDs or biologics.

Medications available: Tofacitinib/ Xeljanz, Baricitinib/ Olumniant, Upadacitinib/ Rinvoq.

Risks: Increased risk of infections (most of the time, upper respiratory infections, otitis, sinusitis, and skin infections, more rare, severe infections), increased risk of herpes virus reactivation (I always recommend zoster virus vaccination before starting therapy) are risks of these medications. There is a recent FDA black box warning I'd like to make you aware of: Those with a history of cardiovascular diseases like strokes or pulmonary emboli are to avoid treatment with JAK inhibitors due to the increasing risk of thrombosis.[15,16]

○ **PROTIP**

If you have a history of heart disease, stroke or pulmonary emboli, is probably best to avoid JAK inhibitors.

Rituximab

This is a potent drug used in patients who don't respond to any of the medications mentioned above or in patients with a recent history of cancer (in the last five years), as no other drugs are allowed. This is the most potent and 'last resort' therapy that can help patients but comes with significant side effects.

Risks: Severe anemia, low platelets, low white blood cells, increased risk of infections, infusion-related reactions.

These are the most common treatments used and prescribed today. Each has its own benefits and risks, and might seem a little scary, the decision to treat RA with any of these drugs must be balanced against the equally scary effects of not using these kinds of treatments. I also want to assure you that there's hope, because cientists are constantly developing novel RA treatments with fewer and fewer side effects.

For example, recently, in 2023, promising research about CAR (stands for Chimeric Antigen Receptor) T cell therapy has emerged. Unlike other therapies, CAR T cell therapy kills inflammatory B cells in the body and re-establishes health in autoimmune organs.[17] Stem cell-based therapies, promising in many forms of medicine, are another effective therapy emerging for RA; these have been proven to reduce proinflammatory marker levels and suppress the immune system response in those struggling with RA.[18] While both of these treatments are in their testing stages, each illustrates a grain of hope I wish to impart to you as you read: There are promising treatments everywhere, some in the form of medication and others in changes you can make on your own. Continue reading to learn more about all of the options available to you.

What Isn't RA?

John was a 52-year-old man who presented as overweight and had a history of hypertension (high blood pressure). When he went to his PCP, he complained of foot pain and swelling in his toes. His doctor ordered laboratory tests and found that his uric acid levels were mildly elevated at about 7 mg/dl (for reference, less than 6 mg/dl is considered 'normal'). He concluded that John most likely suffered from gout and put him on appropriate anti-inflammatory medication and another medication called allopurinol to decrease his uric acid levels. He told him to return in three months for repeat labs and sent John on his way.

This wasn't the end of John's story, however. John continued to struggle with pain and swelling in his foot throughout those three months despite taking his medications as prescribed. Some days weren't so bad, but on others, he was in so much pain that he struggled to walk; the swelling was so intense that he couldn't put on his shoes in the morning.

John returned to the doctor and told him things weren't improving—at least, not quickly. His doctor prescribed him two weeks of prednisone, a much more potent anti-inflammatory and steroid medication. He also increased his allopurinol dosage, thinking that this would help the so-called gout become more controlled.

Those two weeks were bliss for John—he felt like a new man! His swelling had decreased significantly, and he could walk normally again. However, when the prednisone stopped, his pain and swelling returned in full force. He went back to his PCP, and he referred him to a specialist—me.

I listened to John's story and noticed the swelling in his feet was pronounced and severe. By this time, the swelling had spread to his hands, but they weren't nearly as painful as his feet were, so he hadn't mentioned them to his doctor. I ran the necessary tests and X-rays and diagnosed John with RA—not gout, as his PCP had believed.

Often, like John experienced, and historically, there has been a great deal of confusion regarding RA, particularly in the context of other diseases and forms of arthritis. My goal is to give you a brief introduction to these to dispel any concerns you may have and to provide you with a clear look at how (and why) these conditions are separate from Rheumatoid arthritis.

Gout and RA

While some of the symptoms of gout and RA are similar—John's story was an example of this—the two are drastically different ailments and require different treatment approaches.

Unlike RA, an autoimmune disease, gout is a metabolic disease resulting from a buildup of uric acid. Uric acid is created when our body breaks down purine, an organic compound that is naturally occuring in our bodies, but is also derived from certain high-protein foods (e.g., red meat, shellfish, organ meats) as well as alcohol and sugary drinks Typically, our bodies get rid of uric acid when we urinate or have a bowel movement. But when the body can't keep up with the amount of uric acid produced, the buildup leads to gout, kidney stones, or even tophi (uric acid deposits in the skin).

Gout predominantly affects men. That isn't to say that everyone who develops gout is male—women around menopausal age (50s and 60s) are at risk for gout, too. Both diseases are heavily influenced by genetics and lifestyle choices (eating a lot of red meat, drinking alcohol and sugary drinks, for example), and obesity can be a risk factor in both.

Both gout and RA affect your large and small joints and cause pain, swelling, and stiffness. However, most commonly, gout causes excruciating pain in the patient's big toe.

RA vs Lupus

Lupus is an autoimmune disease that affects your entire body, including your joints, muscles, skin, and brain. RA and Lupus have many overlapping symptoms, so understanding the specific characteristics of each is essential to obtaining the correct diagnosis.

What are the common signs of Lupus?
- **Butterfly-shaped facial rash**
- **Increased sensitivity to sun exposure**
- **Oral ulcerations**
- **Joint pain and swelling** affecting the small joints of the hands and feet or other larger joints (shoulders, knees, hips).
- **Fatigue and low-grade fever** lupus patients can present with a low-grade fever, usually at night, accompanied by feeling unwell, tired, or exhausted.
- **Chest pain and shortness of breath**
- **Kidney involvement:** red, frothy, or bubbly urine
- **Neurological symptoms** include headaches, seizures, loss of consciousness, inflammation in the spine, and even tingling and numbness in their hands or feet.
- **Hair loss (alopecia)**
- **Anemia, low white blood cell counts, and low platelet counts**

At first glance, both Rheumatoid arthritis (RA) and lupus share a few key similarities, especially in terms of joint, skin, lung, and blood counts. Yet, they have some distinguishing features: Lupus typically more strongly affects the skin, whereas joint swelling is more common in RA patients. Unlike RA, the damage lupus causes to joints is generally reversible.

RA vs. Psoriatic Arthritis

Psoriatic Arthritis is an inflammatory autoimmune disease that usually occurs in those with psoriasis, a skin condition. Thirty percent of psoriasis patients develop psoriatic arthritis. In most cases, the condition develops about ten years after the onset of skin symptoms.

The most common signs of Psoriatic Arthritis include joint pain (typically worse in the mornings), joint redness and swelling, limited range of motion, loss of function over time, and nail and eye changes.

Psoriatic arthritis occurs asymmetrically, unlike RA, most commonly affecting the knees, fingers, toes, neck, and lower back. There is no cure for psoriatic arthritis, but the symptoms it causes can be managed with medication and lifestyle shifts.

RA vs. Sjogren's

Sjogren's Disease (previously named Sjogren's Syndrome) is a complex autoimmune disorder that can occur independently or alongside other autoimmune conditions like Rheumatoid arthritis, autoimmune liver disease (Primary Biliary Cirrhosis), or Autoimmune Thyroiditis.

About half of individuals with Sjogren's disease experience joint and muscle pain, and it affects both large and small joints. Unlike RA, however, joint inflammation doesn't usually accompany severe swelling or deformities.

Symptoms of Sjogren's
- Dryness in the eyes and mouth
- Extreme fatigue
- Lung disease
- Muscle pain
- Joint pain
- Neurological issues (e.g., from numbness and tingling in the hands or feet to brain damage)

The symptoms of Sjorgren's disease are more neurological, though there is some overlap with RA.

Both conditions affect joints in the hands, wrists, and knees, leading to dangerous lung complications such as fibrosis and breathing issues. However, untreated RA causes joint deformities, while Sjogren's disease doesn't: Patients with Sjogren's disease show damage to other parts of the body, including the eyes, mouth, lungs, nervous system, and brain.

Confusion regarding your symptoms is entirely normal, so I encourage patients not to Google them! Even trained physicians with years of experience treating and managing patients with RA, as was the case with our patient John, can get the diagnosis wrong from time to time. I provide this information not to scare you but to inform you: If you're currently uncertain about your diagnosis, I highly encourage you to seek care from a doctor who can help you discern which diagnosis is right for you.

Hope For Your Future

When I diagnose patients with RA, I receive one of two very different responses: In some cases—about 50%—of patients are relieved. When I deliver what I feel is important news, I approach them with empathy, and, in these cases, I'm greeted with a smile, a sigh of relief, or even a hug. These patients finally have an answer to their question—*what's wrong with me*—and feel grateful for a diagnosis.

However, other patients, when I share the news of their diagnosis, burst into tears, grow angry, or, in some cases, blame themselves. I feel for these patients: They feel RA is an effective death sentence—a clanging knoll on their previously RA-free life. They're worried about the changes they'll have to make, the steps they'll need to take, and the life they feel they can no longer live.

If you've recently received the news of an RA diagnosis and have this response, I want to share with you what I share with all of my patients:

RA, like heart disease, diabetes, or high blood pressure, is a condition, not a label.

The responsible thing to do is understand your condition, accept it, take your treatment, and incorporate all the lifestyle changes I suggest in this book. Be positive, and you will get better.

The information presented in this chapter sounds scary, but I don't want you to fear: You and millions of other people suffer from this disease. You are all in the same boat, so you're the furthest thing from alone.

RA treatment requires a personalized approach, and medication, diet, supplementation, sleep, etc., don't operate as a one-size-fits-all solution. Just like you can change your habits to prevent RA, there are many lifestyle changes you can make after diagnosis to help you cope with and treat your disease.

Throughout this book, we'll uncover the truth behind the diet, the gut-mind connection, lifestyle (including sleep and mindfulness), and movement to help you understand how your behaviors impact your mind, body, and subsequently, your RA. Action steps proven effective will help you easily incorporate manageable changes into your life, leading to an overall less painful outcome.

It's time to take charge of your diagnosis—the steps and information provided in this book will improve you and your life.

CHAPTER 4

TRUST YOUR GUT

What does your gut have to do with Rheumatoid arthritis? In truth, a lot.

In the previous chapters, we explored RA in-depth, discussing who's at risk, how it develops, similar ailments, and standard drug treatments. In this section, we'll take a bit of a detour to discuss a topic that's received a lot of recent traction: the gut microbiome and its role in the development and progression of Rheumatoid arthritis.

Humans Don't Run the World—Bugs Do

In the last ten years, a great deal of emerging information has shifted the public's attention to—you guessed it—the gut microbiome. When I refer to the gut, I'm referring to the organs in your digestive tract: the small and large colon, etc.

Humans are a little self-absorbed. We think humans dominate the world and are responsible for nearly everything happening to and on our planet. Though there's a case for this, the truth is that we're relatively new here, and humans are numerically inferior to the number of microorganisms that have resided in our world for 3.5 billion years.

What is the microbiome?

The microbiome is the collection of microbes, such as bacteria, fungi, viruses, and their genes, that naturally live in our gut.

Like it or not, we're surrounded and inhabited by trillions of bacteria. Our bodies are comprised of roughly 30 trillion human cells, which co-exist with about 38 trillion bacteria on our skin and over 100 trillion microbes in the gut.[1,2] This astounding number can be broken down into between 500 and 1,000 different microbial species, all of whom call your gut their home.

The gut is your body's largest interface between what's inside of you and the world outside. Inside is a vast ecosystem: Picture it like an extensive network of highways in a big city. From a bird's-eye perspective, each of the tiny cars rolling along, stopping at stop signs, and occasionally honking at one another represents a single bacterium (or a single fungi, virus, or parasite) inside your body.

It sounds a little gross, but it's anything but—your gut microbiome is entirely natural. At birth, your body is exposed to tiny microorganisms during delivery or through your mother's breast milk for the first time. Environmental exposures and diet are the main factors affecting our microbiome as we age.

So, what's in your gut microbiome and what's not is determined by your life experiences and the food you consume daily.[3] Just as no two people are identical, no two people's gut microbiomes are identical. In his book *Fiber Fueled,* Dr. Will Bulsiewicz says, "Your gut microbiome is as unique as your fingerprint."[4] Even the gut microbiomes of identical twins aren't the same. You can consume the same food or live in the same space as another person, and your gut microbiome will still differ from theirs.

As we humans are unique, the gut microbiome is unique to us. In other words, each human carries a unique combination of gut microbes.

The Microbial 'Engine'

But what does the gut microbiome do? The short answer? Many things. Humans and our gut bacteria are deeply connected, relying on one another for many tasks and duties. In *Fiber Fueled,* Dr. Bulsiewicz compares the gut microbiome to a factory staffed by tiny workers, our gut microbes. These tiny employees are responsible for operating and managing many of our body's essential functions, like immunity, hormone regulation, metabolism (or the digestion of food), cognition, and gene expression.

It's difficult to understand the magnitude of these gut microbes on our health, but scientists liken it to our engine, which isn't an exaggeration. Just like you can't operate a car without an engine, you can't live without your gut microbiome—that's how important it is.

The gut microbiome is like a 'second brain' because it's constantly conversing with the mind. In other words, what's going on in your mind directly correlates with what's happening in the gut. It sounds a bit wild, but whether you're awake, asleep, working, napping, or doing something, the two are busy influencing one another.

How do they hold that conversation? How do they talk to each other? The brain and the gut communicate via the vagus nerve. The vagus nerve is one of the longest and most complex cranial nerves, connecting your brain to your heart, lungs, and gut, sending messages in both directions. Think of it as a sort of messenger—it's through this nerve that chronic stress influences the gut microbiome.

Neurotransmitters, substances used by your brain to control emotions, feelings, and sensations, send signals through the vagus nerve from the brain to other parts of the body, including the gut. For example, serotonin, the body's 'happy' hormone, is one of these neurotransmitters. You've likely heard of serotonin before, but I bet you didn't know that your gut microbiome produces 95% of your body's serotonin. It travels to your brain via the vagus nerve, making you happy. Literally and figuratively, keeping the gut happy keeps the brain happy!

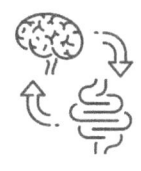

> **Did you know?** Your gut microbiome is deeply connected with your brain, immune system cells, pain sensation, hormone production, and expression of your genes.

And while the gut microbiome can make us happy, it can influence other emotions, like sadness, depression, and, most prominently, anxiety. Think about the last time you grew nervous about something. It's likely that, when you did, you felt the flutter of tiny butterflies in your stomach. These butterflies aren't real, actual butterflies; this feeling is caused by—you guessed it—the gut microbiome. Your stress levels influence your gut microbiome.[5]

Just like the gut microbiome influences happiness and stress, it can also influence pain. Specific metabolites that are produced by gut microbiome activate pathways that lead to and cause pain, connecting your brain with the heart, lungs, and gut, sending messages in both directions. One study on RA patients found that activating the vagus nerve naturally through singing, deep breathing, laughing, or electrical stimulation reduces pain or eliminates it altogether.[6] That said, the messaging system between the gut and the brain holds significant weight in how, if, and when your body functions.

The Body's Second Immune System

The gut microbiome performs various necessary functions, including mood regulation, digestion, hormone transmission, and, most importantly, immune health for RA patients.

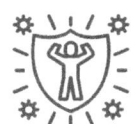

Your gut is lined with immune system cells whose 'job' is to detect pathogens, or things that might hurt you. In fact, the immune cells in your gut represent 70% of your immune system, responsible for fighting infection and even detecting potentially cancerous cells. Throughout the day (and night), these microbes defend the gut from the invasion of disease-causing bacteria—they're your body's first line of defense from the outside world. Your gut's immune cells, that are lining just below your gut mucosae, are constantly conversing with your gut microbiome, and the two are quite chatty, constantly speaking to one another.

A mucus shield protects this gut lining, constantly maintaining the barrier between your body's cells and the microbes inside your gut. So, the lining itself serves two functions:

1. Shield the body's cells from what's inside the gut and,
2. The gut lining becomes food for the microbiome if the microbes aren't fed appropriately.

The gut microbiome is so powerful that it moderates the magnitude and duration of your body's immune system response, ensuring it's going at the right pace. But sometimes, the conversation occurring between the two can become a little loud: For example, if the body's immune defense is too strong, gut microbes launch an excessive attack, causing too much inflammation and increasing your risk for autoimmune diseases. If it comes on too slowly, the pathogenic bacteria win the battle, causing an infection.

The conversation between your microbiome and your immune cells is crucial. When their 'conversation' is going well, or when your gut bacteria is balanced and healthy, your immune system is likely to be too. In individuals with healthy guts (and, thus, a healthy gut microbiome), gut microorganisms can fight disease and prevent other unwelcome ailments.

That said, your gut isn't just a collection of cells whose job is to absorb and digest the food you eat. Rather, it's the home of both your gut microbiome and your body's immune cells; these cells interact with one another to either protect you from disease or increase your risk of developing one.

Living In Harmony: The Impact of Microbial Dysbiosis

Some gut microorganisms are (usually) 'good,' while others aren't. 'Good' microorganisms exist in a mutually beneficial symbiotic relationship with your body, helping and fueling functions you need to survive. 'Bad' bacteria, or pathogenic bacteria, on the other hand, isn't so good. Harmful bacteria can promote disease and cause issues in bodily functioning.

In healthy people, good and bad bacteria live in harmony, sending positive signals to each other and the rest of the body. If we think back to the traffic example, we understand this to be the steady flow of cars, trucks, and vehicles, all moving down an extensive road and behaving as expected. However, this balance and harmony can go haywire: When there are too many harmful bacteria in the gut, or when our gut doesn't have enough diversity in microbial species, this balance is disrupted, causing potential health issues. Disruption of this balance is called *dysbiosis*.

Dysbiosis, or the imbalance in your gut microbiome, is caused by several factors, including illness, poor diet, or medication overuse. Cultural changes and shifts cause all of these. Over the last few hundred years, our culture has changed dramatically. Today, we live mostly indoors: We often sit on the couch, drink soda, and order food through online apps that deliver it right to our door. Our diet is highly processed and full of sugar, salt, and fat. Many of our meals are pre-cooked—all we have to do is put them in the microwave. We clean our surfaces with chemicals, wash our hands extensively, and apply sanitizers multiple times daily. We don't allow our children to pick things off floors or play outside in the creek or the mud, but we allow them to play video games for hours in the house.

So—what are the consequences? As I previously noted, along with our environment, diet plays a significant role in determining which helpful and harmful bacteria live in your intestine (small and big intestine). The high-fat, high-sugar, low-fiber Western diet starves our gut bacteria.[7] Without proper nutrients, your gut bacteria search for food elsewhere and begin eating the mucus of your gut lining, damaging it. This damage causes the lining to leak toxic metabolites into your bloodstream (commonly known as "leaky gut"), causing inflammation and increasing the risk of autoimmune conditions.

However, a high-fiber diet increases the amount of "good" bacteria that live in the colon (we'll discuss fiber in more depth in Chapter 5). This is just one example; we'll cover the specific foods, actions, and supplements that positively and negatively impact gut health later in this book.

Besides diet, excessive use of medications, over-the-counter or prescription, affects your gut microbiome. In recent years, the number of Americans using medications has increased drastically: Three out of five American (about 130 million) adults use prescription medications.[8] 270 million antibiotic prescriptions are filled annually in the United States–these antibiotics deplete the number of good bacteria species in your gut. Plus, more than 30 million Americans use over-the-counter non-steroidal medications (NSAIDs) like ibuprofen or naproxen every day. Unfortunately, NSAIDs alter the gut microbiome and destroy your intestinal lining, causing ulcerations, which will increase gut inflammation and also boost your risk of developing Inflammatory bowel diseases like Crohn's disease, Ulcerative colitis, or microscopic colitis.

> **What are the most common medications that affect your gut microbiome?**
>
> Antibiotics and NSAIDs like ibuprofen, naproxen and diclofenac.

Did you know that just a few days of antibiotic use wipes out 50% of your gut microbiome?[9] Such a loss is difficult to recover from; it takes months or years to recover the bacteria lost. Antibiotic use can cause some bacteria in the gut microbiome to develop resistance, and other species may disappear entirely.

○ **PROTIP**

Talk to your doctor before taking any medication, and ask yourself, "Do you really need it?"

These significant changes force our gut microbiome into survival mode. They constantly adapt to their new environment, battling severe challenges that threaten their existence. Unfortunately, many good bacteria disappear entirely during this battle, while other potentially bad bacteria thrive and overgrow in number. This process causes lower gut diversity, or dysbiosis.

Unfortunately, scientists across the world are already watching this happen: The average American adult has approximately 1,200 different microbial species living in their gut, while adults living in less industrialized areas, such as Venezuela, have over 1,600 bacteria species in their gut.[10]

This is a glaring problem: Lower gut diversity equates to a higher incidence of autoimmune diseases. Because the number of bacterial species in our guts is decreasing so dramatically, scientists have observed an increase in the number of individuals diagnosed with autoimmune diseases like lupus, for which rates have multiplied threefold.[11] We're also experiencing a rise in cases of inflammatory bowel disease, Rheumatoid arthritis, and other autoimmune diseases.[12]

> *Lower gut diversity equates to a higher incidence of autoimmune diseases.*

Widespread dysbiosis leaves us at risk for an epidemic of chronic conditions like asthma, food allergies, Crohn's disease, obesity, and, guess what—autoimmune diseases like Rheumatoid arthritis, Lupus, Ankylosing spondylitis, and many others.

Go With Your Gut: RA, Dysbiosis, and the Gut Microbiome

What does RA have to do with all of this? How does dysbiosis cause RA? Now that we understand the vital role of your body's tiny microbes in your overall health, it's time to zoom in a little further.

Dysbiosis is a major cause for concern for RA patients. Microbial imbalances throughout your body can negatively impact or even cause your disease.

Interestingly, dysbiosis doesn't begin in the gut but in the mouth. For example, *Porphyromonas gingivalis,* a type of oral bacteria, has been linked to an increased risk of developing RA. This is the same bacteria that causes gingivitis, gum disease, and periodontal disease, called periodontitis, an inflammatory oral disease. Periodontitis is more prevalent in RA patients when compared to the general population, and patients can suffer from periodontitis for years before they develop RA. Furthermore, both periodontitis and RA destroy bone: Peridontitis causes erosion of the bone surrounding your teeth, resulting in tooth loss.

Recent research connects these two diseases. While RA negatively impacts periodontitis, peridontitis aggravates your RA.[13] It's believed that the bacteria causing oral dysbiosis stimulate the immune system, likely leading to RA onset.

Moving down the digestive tract, in 2022, scientists found a new bacteria called Subdoligranulum Didolesgii in the feces of RA patients.[14] Oddly enough, this bacteria was absent in those who didn't suffer from RA, indicating that changes in the gut microbiome can cause and influence who develops RA and who doesn't.

This isn't the only bacteria linked to RA. Unfortunately, certain bad bacterial species, like Colinsella, Prevotella copri, are more prevalent in RA patients.[15] Scientists speculate that these bacteria increase mucosal permeability, causing "leaky gut syndrome." Tears in the gut lining leave the immune system constantly stimulated and on guard, causing autoimmunity and RA.

While we're just scratching the surface of understanding how and why the gut microbiome causes chronic diseases, we can't ignore this information.

These studies establish a link between the gut microbiome and who develops, but what about patients already diagnosed with RA? Recently, promising studies indicate that our gut microbes can help alleviate patient symptoms, with certain good bacteria helping slow the progression of RA.[16]

In patients like you who are currently suffering from RA, starting a medication regimen of methotrexate can help restore your gut microbiome.[17] However, as we've discussed, not all medications positively impact gut microbes, so less medication is usually the better option.[18]

Because of this, you can't rely solely on medication to solve your symptoms. Lifestyle changes are the best way to fix these issues. Your gut microbiome is heavily regulated by the foods you eat, mood changes, sleep, and stress levels. So, while medication may be necessary, lifestyle changes will make your treatment plan more effective.

For example, a 2022 study found that a 'supercharged' diet of foods commonly eaten by those living around the Mediterranean Sea profoundly changed the patient's gut microbiome in only two weeks.[19] As we'll discuss in more depth later in the next Chapter, the Mediterranean diet consists of whole grains, low red meat consumption, leafy green vegetables, green juices, oily fish, nuts, and avocado, among other nutritious foods.

The result?

Patients who followed the diet showed a profound change in their gut microbes and experienced less pain and inflammation. This is among the first studies to illustrate the effects of diet and the gut microbiome on RA patients, and as a doctor, I'm compelled by these results.

Speaking firsthand, I've noticed that patients who follow a healthy, anti-inflammatory diet report less pain and fewer RA symptoms than those who don't.

This is excellent news for you: Because our diet influences our gut microbiome, these studies indicate the value of actionable dietary interventions for pain and symptoms.

It All Comes Back To Lifestyle

As discussed in this chapter, the gut microbiome is much more important than you might initially believe. Not only do these tiny organisms impact digestion, mood, and other crucial body functions, but dysbiosis, or disruption to this balance, can play a pivotal role in the development and maintenance of RA.

Your gut microbiome, immune system, and how you feel are profoundly interconnected and balanced—changes in one of these cause changes in another. Your diet and the foods you regularly eat are the key factors determining the microbiome's balance of good bacteria versus harmful bacteria, which can impact pain and inflammation levels. Keeping this bacteria happy is crucial because of its integral role in your immune system.

 Medications, cultural shifts, and the unhealthy foods we regularly eat each shift this balance, and not for the better. In this book, we address all lifestyle choices that change your gut microbiome, leading to less inflammation and pain.

As you're starting to see, there are many, many ways to manage your RA symptoms, and not all of them are pills or expensive drugs. Diet and lifestyle changes can alter and impact your pain and symptoms as effectively as medication can, sometimes cutting your reliance on medication entirely.

As I often say, you are the CEO of your RA, and even when you feel hope is lost, you can still make changes to get better. Let's pay attention to our lifestyle, from what we eat, which medications we take, how much we sleep, and how much stress we endure.

CHAPTER 5

NUTRITION 101: DETOXIFY, HEAL, AND SUPERCHARGE

We've established that diet is critical to your Rheumatoid arthritis treatment plan. But we haven't yet answered the questions, "What should I avoid?" and "What should I eat?"

In this chapter, I'll give you the low-down on foods proven to cause inflammation, those shown to lessen it, and those that will supercharge your diet.

Starting a diet can be overwhelming, especially when you're also navigating persistent inflammation, fatigue, and pain. To that end, we'll use a simple, stepwise approach to help you through the process. Consider this chapter's three parts: detoxification, heal, and supercharge, like you would cleaning up a dirty kitchen. The process takes work, dedication, and healthy lifestyle changes, but the result is a clean space, or in this case, a body free of inflammation, fatigue, and pain. In other words, while you might feel a little overwhelmed at first, the payoff is completely worth it!

Imagine walking into a dirty kitchen for the first time—and I mean dirty. You notice old wrappers and food waste all over the floor, in the cabinets, and littering the space's nooks and crannies. The space is in complete disarray, and you don't know where or how to begin cleaning things up and making it livable.

First, we'll talk about **detoxification**. Detoxification is picking up all the clutter littering a dirty kitchen–it is the crucial process of eliminating harmful foods from your routine. This step is pivotal to clearing out the debris harming your immune system. There's no sense in wiping off a counter covered in old food, right?

After we get rid of the clutter, or in this case, the food-related toxins stopping you from reclaiming your life, we can move on to some deep cleaning. But you have know the right way to clean. Anyone who's ever cleaned a kitchen knows the importance of choosing the right cleaning supplies to eliminate unwanted dust and grime. Bleach wipes on wooden surfaces can damage them, leaving peeling varnish in their wake. But bleach wipes used on a grimy sink work wonders. In the **heal** section, we'll discuss which nutrients re-balance your gut and foods that revive your immune system and fight inflammation.

Finally, after you've cleaned out the clutter (detoxified) and deep cleaned (started healing) , we can begin the **supercharge** process. I'll introduce compelling nutrition regimens like Mediterranean and vegetarian diets, which are proven to combat inflammation and pain in RA patients. I'll also provide my re-designed RA-friendly food pyramid to guide your journey. In short, the **supercharge** section gives you an organized approach to the nutrition knowledge we discussed in previous sections.

When we're finished, just like when you're done cleaning, your body will be much like a clean house—fresh and ready to make your life and RA symptoms more manageable.

Throughout the chapter, I'll tell you a few stories about those who've completed these steps, and we'll talk about the science behind each in case you need a little extra convincing. Furthermore, we'll discuss specific, practical changes you can make to get yourself and your RA back on track. Each section will provide concrete and practical action steps to start your diet-friendly RA journey.

I encourage you to take these steps with me: You, your brain, and your body will thank me later!

Detoxification 101

It's time to get rid of pesky debris and prepare for a deep clean! In this section, we'll cover which foods, and nutrients to eliminate and, most importantly, how. Let's begin together.

Sugar

Thomas was a 42-year-old gentleman who'd been diagnosed with RA three years before this conversation occurred. He was slightly overweight and suffered from high blood pressure and type 2 diabetes. Thomas told me that he was taking his medication diligently and that, while he felt a little better than he had before, he didn't feel like his old self again just yet.

"My joints feel a little bit better, but I don't know why I'm so tired all the time," he said, a little confused. During this conversation, Thomas explained that he had some mild pain in his feet each day and that he was battling overall feelings of exhaustion despite getting plenty of sleep. "My tests look great, but my body says otherwise. What else can I do?"

"Well," I began. "Let's talk briefly about your diet and how to make changes."

"Can I change my diet?" he looked at me, perplexed, just as many patients are when they first hear this news.

"Yes–you can," I told him. "Let's start with a food diary. Record everything you eat and drink for the next two weeks. When you come back, we can talk about it."

Thomas did just that, and two weeks later, we began reviewing his diet. I noticed that Thomas was drinking 1-2 cans of soda with each meal. I looked at him and asked, "How much water do you drink daily?"

"Not so much," he replied. "But I drink coffee, iced tea, and sodas to keep myself hydrated."

"Here's the issue, Thomas," I said, sitting beside him. "The soda you're drinking contains lots of sugar, which could be making you feel so tired and achy. Let's start with the soda—that's a small change."

Sugar, ordinarily in drinks like soda, is the generic name for anything that tastes sweet. Sugar can be broken down into simple sugars, like glucose, fructose, lactose (monosaccharides), and compound sugars, which are just two simple sugar molecules combined. Sucrose, or table sugar, is an example; sucrose consists of one glucose and one fructose molecule linked together. Beyond these, there are more complex forms of sugars, such as starch, a glucose polymer commonly found in plants.

Artificial vs natural sugars

Natural forms of sugar
- Honey and fruits (Fructose)
- Dairy (Lactose)
- Sugar cane and beets (Sucrose)

Artificial forms of sugar
- High fructose corn syrup (HFCS)
- Aspartame (NutraSweet, Equal)
- Saccharin (Sweet'N Low)
- Sucralose (Splenda)

Natural or artificial sugars are often added to beverages, ultra-processed foods, sweetened breakfast cereals, and even bread or ham.

The average American consumes 57 pounds of sugar yearly, ten times more than 100 years ago. As Thomas noticed, this isn't a good thing—not in the slightest.

Most of us eat 300% more sugar than is recommended, but why is this the case?[1] Unfortunately, the blame rests on the food industry. Sugar manipulates your taste buds into thinking food tastes better, so you become addicted to it and keep buying.

In the 1960s and 1970s, manufacturers began adding sugar to anything and everything to boost revenue. They launched a nationwide campaign dispelling sugar's negative consequences on our health, and the public bought it, literally and figuratively. Added sugar is a gimmick—one we fall for daily.

Though they're quite tasty, sugar serves another purpose: It's a 'natural' preservative, capable of lengthening the time a food can sit in a display at the grocery store or atop your shelf, increasing its marketability.

> ○ **PROTIP**
>
> Food manufacturing companies use various names when referring to sugar, including sucrose, glucose, fructose, or maltose, to hide that they're using too much of it. When you look for the food labels for the nutritional content, anything with an *-ose* at the end is likely sugar.

Furthermore, sugar-rich foods can cause insulin spikes, making you hungrier. Thomas was an example of this: Repeatedly, he fell for the added sugar trap, causing him to eat more, run out of it faster, and head back to the store and buy more.

The problem is this: There's a significant difference between *manufactured* sugar, the sugar *naturally* found in fruits and vegetables, and how each affects your health. Plenty of research corroborates this, but I'll share with you one study. Research from the UK found that beverages and foods teacoffee, and cereals, when they are sweetened with sugar, are associated with high blood sugar, weight gain, type 2 diabetes, heart disease, and, importantly, higher markers of inflammation.[2,3] However, sugar from fruit, vegetables, and dairy products—or natural sugars—didn't yield similar results.

It's safe to say that natural sugars don't do the same damage to our bodies as processed or manufactured sugar does, meaning it's safe to continue consuming sugar from fruits and whole foods.

Excess sugar intake is associated with
- Obesity
- Type 2 diabetes
- Fatty liver disease
- Heart disease
- Tooth decay
- Alzheimer's disease and other cognitive ailments
- Cancer

High Fructose Corn Syrup (HFCS)

HFCS is just one of many examples of these dangerous manufactured sugars. It is a man-made sweetener from corn starch, usually containing 55% fructose and 45% glucose. HFCS is relatively cheap to produce, and because the food industry's goal is to make money, HFCS is commonly added to our baked goods, soft drinks, energy drinks, and other ultra-processed foods. Generally, products high in HFCS are also often high in unhealthy fats and salt and low in fiber.

Here's the kicker: Excessive consumption of products high in HFCS can cause fructose to build up in the body. Fructose needs to be processed and metabolized by the liver, but large amounts cause the liver to go into hyperdrive. After a while, the liver experiences what can only be referred to as 'burnout,' causing non-alcoholic fatty liver disease and an increase of uric acid in the body (which, as we discussed in Chapter 3, leads to gout).[4]

HFCS disastrously damages the liver but can also lead to inflammation, type 2 diabetes, and even cancer.[5]

Not all fructose is bad for you!

There's a big difference between consuming fructose from HCFS and consuming it through fruits. In addition to fructose, fruits contain fiber and other nutrients, slowing fructose metabolism. In short, eating fruit doesn't cause non-alcoholic fatty liver disease, while HFCS consumption does.

Sugar & Rheumatoid arthritis

Unfortunately, research links excessive sugar consumption with autoimmune diseases like Rheumatoid arthritis, Psoriasis, Autoimmune thyroiditis, and Ulcerative Colitis. While the exact cause of this isn't entirely understood, scientists believe that the issue lies in the fact that foods high in sugar are often low in fiber. As we briefly noted in Chapter 4, fiber is food for our gut microbiome. Without it, the microbiome starves, and good bacteria die out, leaving a breeding ground for harmful bacteria to flourish. These hungry bacteria eat through the gut lining and enter the bloodstream, ready to cause even more damage. Because of this, excessive sugar intake causes inflammation and autoimmunity, priming your body for autoimmune conditions like RA.

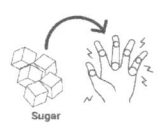

Additionally, as we'll discuss later in this chapter, a low fiber intake yields a lower production of short-chain fatty acids (SCFAs), the metabolites responsible for reducing inflammation in the body. For those suffering from RA, SCFAs are crucial, and without them, the body remains in a constant state of inflammation and high disease activity. In simpler terms, few SCFAs cause more swelling, inflammation, and fatigue.

> ○ **PROTIP**
>
> **Sugar-Free Foods aren't any better. Aspartame use was linked to changes in the microbiome, diabetes, more inflammation, and more pain.**

Here's the facts: Sugar doesn't just exacerbate RA, but causes it. One study examined over 100,000 women over 20 years, finding that those who drank more than one can of soda each day were at 63% higher risk for developing RA.[6] Soda drinkers were also at higher risk for developing more severe forms of the condition, and for women over the age of 55, drinking more than one can of soda per day increases your risk of developing RA by 2.64—over double.

While I *can't* say that Thomas's condition was caused by his soda consumption, I *can* say that it didn't help. I do believe, however, that soda was worsening his RA, and studies support this. One survey of different foods consumed by RA patients found that those who drank more sugary drinks or ate more desserts reported worsening symptoms in the days that followed.[7]

Let's go back to Thomas's story: Gradually, over the coming months, Thomas replaced soda with glasses of water, still allowing himself the occasional can when dining out.

> O **PROTIP**
>
> **Drinking soda every day increases your risk of developing RA.**

The transformation was evident: He returned to me a few months later and reported feeling more energetic—his steps felt much lighter. At this appointment, he told me, "I never realized such a small change could make such a big difference. I feel like a different man!"

Thomas's story serves as a reminder of the harsh effects of sugar on your body, particularly when you're battling RA. For those already struggling with the disease, manufactured sugar can worsen your symptoms.

The takeaway is clear: For those with RA, decreasing sugar intake can lower overall inflammation, improve gut dysbiosis, increase energy levels, and reduce fatigue and pain. Start by reducing the amount of sugar you eat and tracking your symptoms.

How to reduce sugar in your day?

ACTION STEPS

1. Go to your pantry and empty all sugar containers, including sugar bags, cookies, and candies.
2. When you cook, reduce the sugar suggested in your recipes by half. Try to replace sugar with honey, stevia, or monk fruit. Avoid artificial sweeteners (e.g., aspartame) at all costs.
3. At the grocery store, be a detective! Look for HFCS and sugar substitutes on food labels.
4. Replace your sugar-sweetened beverages with still or mineral water. Gradually reduce the amount of sugar you add to your coffee and tea each week.
5. Cut back on the soda you consume—start by cutting one can a week, and go from there until you replace it all. You can have soda just on rare occasions.

Salt

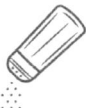

Much like sugar, salt is found in many foods on our shelves. Salt acts as a flavor enhancer, meaning that foods with high amounts taste just a little bit better than those without. Unfortunately, excessive salt consumption is linked to cancer, heart disease, and Rheumatoid arthritis.

Salt is particularly disastrous for your health. High-salt diets cause inflammation by manipulating our immune cell's natural function.[8] When they detect excessive inflammation, T-regulatory cells suppress the body's immune response, calming it down to avoid unnecessary flare ups. Salt inhibits this process, halting these cell's ability to naturally suppress the body's immune response, causing overactive inflammation.

When it comes to people with RA, a recent study published in 2021 showed that excessive salt intake increases joint pain and swelling, as well as hypertension.[9]

Salt is common in many of the foods we eat. It inhibits your immune cell's natural response, making it a 'must not eat' for RA patients. Follow the symptom-busting action steps below to eliminate it.

How do you reduce salt in your day?

ACTION STEPS

1. Head to your table and get rid of your salt shaker. Keep salt in the cupboard only.
2. Remove processed foods (usually high in Salt) from your pantry and fridge, like ham, salami, pre-cooked meals, chips, and fried foods.
3. Replace salt with spices such as garlic, turmeric, cumin, basil, and ginger in recipes.
4. Aim to consume less than salt per day, about one teaspoon (2,300 mg)

Fats & Oils: The Good and The Bad

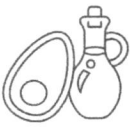

Within the scientific community, the role of fats in, well, fattening is highly debated. Because of this discrepancy, understanding which fats are good and what to eliminate can be confusing to the general public. In this section, we'll cover which fats you should avoid and how these bad fats influence inflammation.

Like many other things, quality and quantity are key in the case of fat. The quality of your fats and the type of fat in your food is similarly vital to how much you consume. In other words, while eating fats doesn't necessarily have a detrimental effect on your body, the type and amount you eat matter.

Some fats are good, while others aren't so much.

Unsaturated fats are—usually—the good kind. These fats are separated into monounsaturated fatty acids (MUFA) and polyunsaturated fatty acids (PUFA). Good fats, or unsaturated fats, are an essential nutrient responsible for many bodily processes, including energy storage and insulating and protecting your internal organs. Good fats also maintain your cell membranes, brain structure, and hormone levels. We'll discuss these more later in the chapter.

Unhealthy fats, like trans fats and saturated fats, are bad. Trans fats, for example, are often present in frozen pizzas, fried foods, and bacon. Trans fats are created through an industrial process called hydrogenation, which adds hydrogen molecules to vegetable oils, making them appear more solid and giving them a more desirable texture and flavor. Trans fats raise your LDL (or *bad*) cholesterol and lower HDL (or *good*) cholesterol, which places you at high risk for heart disease.

Saturated fats are the other 'bad' kind. Common in meat products, high-fat dairy foods (processed cheese and sour cream), and processed foods (such as pizza, hamburgers, desserts, etc.), saturated fats are solid at room temperature because they're fully 'saturated' with hydrogen molecules, meaning they can cluster together and must be warmed to liquefy. Saturated fats are a large contributor to heart disease, obesity, and diabetes, and, in the U.S., we eat too many of them—by a lot. However, when consumed sparingly, small quantities of saturated fats from real butter and small portions of meat products (such as beef from cows fed organic feed) are good for your health.

> Contrary to what marketing tells you, many vegetable oils are similarly unhealthy; many vegetable oils contain solvents to make them shinier and more attractive, but these can cause a range of health issues. On the bottles, these are advertised to support and boost your heart health; nothing is further than the truth! Many vegetable oils (ex. corn, sunflower, and even canola oil) contain an unhealthy balance of omega-6 to omega-3 fats.

Table 1. Good vs Bad Fats

Good Fats	Bad Fats
MUFA • Olives • Olive oil • Nuts (almonds, cashews, pecans) • Avocados	Food with high saturated fats*: • Beef, lamb, pork, poultry, especially with skin • lard and cream • Butter (in excess) • cheese • Palm and Coconut
PUFA (Omega 3s, Omega -6s FA) • Fatty or oily fish (anchovies, herring, mackerel, black cod, salmon, sardines, bluefin tuna, striped bass) • Nuts and seeds, including walnuts, flaxseeds, and sunflower seeds.	Trans Fats • Margarine • Commercial baked goods (cakes, cookies, pies) • Ice cream • Microwave popcorn • Frozen pizza • Refrigerated dough (biscuits and rolls) • Fried foods, doughnuts and fried chicken • Non Dairy coffee creamer

The American Heart Association recommends aiming for a dietary pattern that achieves 5% to 6% of calories from saturated fat (for example, eating about 2,000 calories a day, no more than 120 of them should come from saturated fat).

But what's the risk of consuming unhealthy fats?

Weight gain is certainly one. One study looked at individuals over just two weeks and found that those who consumed a diet of ultra-processed foods gained 0.4 kg, while those who ate a plant-based, minimally processed diet saw weight loss.[10] I find this study's timeframe most interesting—it took only two weeks for the benefits of a plant-based diet to kick into gear!

I don't necessarily promote weight loss in this book, but I must draw your attention to the pertinent relationship between weight gain and RA. Weight 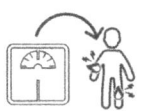 gain and inflammation are deeply connected, and weight can be a precursor for your uncomfortable inflammation.[11] Our body's fat or adipose tissue is an active organ. Throughout the day, adipose tissue secretes hormones and cytokines called adipokines.

Leptin, a hormone linking your body's endocrine system to your immune system, is one of these. Leptin isn't bad on its own. However, the more adipose tissue, or fat, you have, the more adipokines and leptin your body releases. Scientists believe that excess leptin creates more inflammation and causes damage to joint cartilage. And, the more leptin your body releases, the more inflammation and pain you'll experience.

Looking more specifically at RA, studies report that high leptin levels in the blood cause higher disease activity.[12] Furthermore, leptin is associated with increased inflammatory markers, such as Tumor Necrosis Factor (TNF) - alpha, IL-1, and IL-6, which cause cartilage degradation and inhibit bone reabsorption.[13]

In short, an increase in weight can lead to an increase in inflammation, as obesity is a risk factor for RA and other autoimmune diseases. Because unhealthy fats cause weight gain, it's best to eliminate these from your diet.

Are *non-fat* and *low-fat* diets better?

By the 1970s, *non-fat* and *low-fat* diets were popularized by marketing campaigns in the food landscape. However, manufacturers of these foods just replaced the fat with sugar to enhance taste, making these an unhealthy option.

How to choose more of the good fats?

ACTION STEPS

1. Try cooking at home frequently.
2. Cook using a baking, boiling, or convection oven, and avoid frying.
3. Use olive oil daily (e.g., 2-3 tablespoons in your salads)
4. Avoid overeating red meat (beef, lamb, pork)
5. Avoid any processed and pre-cooked food.
6. Eat fatty fish such as tuna and sardines 2-3 times per week.
7. Eat one handful of nuts daily]

Dairy

Dairy isn't always bad, but for RA patients, certain dairy products high in sugar exacerbate inflammation, leading to further joint damage. On one hand, dairy, including milk, yogurt, eggs, and cheese, are potent sources of protein and calcium in your diet. Many fortified dairy products, like milk, contain vitamin D necessary to maintain your body's bones and muscles. Others, like eggs, are low in saturated fat and calories and rich in protein, vitamins, and minerals.

On the other hand, *processed* dairy products may play a role in promoting inflammation: Processed cheese, cheese spreads, flavored and overly sweetened yogurt, and eggs from grain-fed chickens contain harmful amounts of fats, sugar and salt, which cause inflammation. Some people, such as those who suffer from lactose intolerance, are sensitive to certain types of dairy. For these individuals, dairy causes inflammation in the gut that travels to the rest of the body.

> **Do *non-fat* products mean NO fat?**
>
> So-called *fat-free* or *non-fat* products contain less than 0.5 grams of fat per serving, while low-fat foods may have 3 grams of fat or less per serving.

Like fats, some dairy products are better than others: Unprocessed cheeses, like cottage and fermented cheese, eggs from grass-fed chickens, and plain yogurt and kefir, are positive sources of nutrients in your diet. Milk is another example; milk contains essential proteins and nutrients, such as fats and calcium, that benefit your RA in moderate quantities. Some studies support the benefits of drinking milk to prevent osteoarthritis progression, and milk consumption has been shown to reduce arthritis progression in women specifically.[14] More broadly, drinking milk hasn't been shown to impact your risk of developing RA or influence this disease's activity.[15]

While the jury is still out about dairy, eliminating processed cheese, super-flavored yogurt, and eggs from grain-fed chickens is a powerful way to inhibit inflammation and fight pain. Check out the action steps to determine which dairy products you should enjoy, and which you shouldn't.

> **What dairy products are good for you?**
>
> ACTION STEPS
> 1. Consume unprocessed yogurt (Greek yogurt) or kefir each day.
> 2. Look for organic milk and eggs from grass-fed chickens;
> 3. If you are lactose intolerant, replace milk with almond and oat milk!
> 4. Aim to eat 2-3 grass fed chicken egg servings a week (scrambled or hard-boiled)
> 5. Combine yogurt with fresh fruit and chia seeds
> 6. Avoid all processed cheese, cheese spreads, and flavored sweetened yogurt.

Gluten

Similar to fats and dairy, gluten isn't necessarily 'bad' or 'good.' In recent years, diet influencers have flocked from gluten in droves, claiming that it's fattening and 'bad' for your health, but this isn't quite the case for all people and can be confusing.

Gluten is a protein and natural binding agent in many grains, including wheat, barley, and rye. Gluten was first eaten in breads and recipes with wheat flour, and today, it still is— many people eat gluten in breads, cereals, pizzas, pasta, crackers, and desserts. Because of its binding qualities, gluten is also present in some processed meats, medications, and even chewing gum.

Did you know that these products contain gluten?
- Sauces
- Spreads
- Dressings
- Processed meats
- Vegetarian meat substitutes
- Beer
- Malt vinegar
- Playdough
- Some medications
- Some supplements
- Some cosmetics

Is gluten bad or good? For those with a gluten intolerance or gluten sensitivity, gluten is a bad thing, and it all begins in the colon: In the gut, thousands of enzymes break down the food we eat. Protease is just one of these enzymes; its job is to break down the gluten we consume. Those with an intolerance or sensitivity to gluten have a genetic mutation that inhibits these proteases from working correctly, leaving gluten undigested. This undigested gluten causes gut inflammation that affects the lining and triggers an immune response, causing even more systemic inflammation.

Unfortunately, there aren't strong tests available to determine whether or not you're sensitive to gluten. We do, however, have tests for celiac disease, such as a blood test to determine if specific antibodies are present or a small bowel biopsy (though this test can be challenging to obtain). The best test to determine whether or not you're gluten-sensitive or intolerant is to eliminate gluten and track your symptoms.

> ○ **PROTIP**
>
> **The most common signs of gluten sensitivity or intolerance:**
> - Abdominal pain
> - Cramping
> - Bloating
> - Diarrhea
> - Rashes
> - Headaches
> - Joint pain

What about gluten and RA? While gluten may not be the cause of your inflammation, some studies show that those with RA adopting a gluten-free diet benefit from the shift. One study looking at overweight and obese RA patients found that those who removed red meat, gluten, and lactose for three months experienced a substantial reduction in weight and leptin levels.[17] As we discussed in the 'unhealthy fat' section, weight and inflammation go hand in hand: High leptin levels can potentially cause stronger disease activity and symptoms. This study supported these results: Those who adopted a gluten-free diet enjoyed less pain and lower inflammation levels.

> **Did you know?** Celiac disease can mimic RA? Yes, celiac disease may cause joint pain, mild swelling, and morning stiffness in the hands and other joints. Interestingly, in rare cases, RA and celiac disease were reported in the same patient.[16]

The goal is twofold: Consume less gluten, and incorporate more gluten-free whole grains (see the chart below for some examples). Try a gluten-free diet for six months, and maintain a strict diary tracking your symptoms (ex., affected joints, joint swelling, morning stiffness, etc.). Don't expect to notice immediate results; instead, track your symptoms to find gradual changes. If you don't see improvement, consume a diet that includes healthy grains and gluten, and avoid processed foods.

Table 2. Gluten-rich grains vs Gluten-free grains

Gluten-rich grains	Gluten-free grains
• Wheat • Rye • Barley • Wheat berries • Semolina • Durum • Farina • Oats (cross-contamination)	• Quinoa • Brown, black, or red rice • Buckwheat • Amaranth • Corn • Gluten-free oats

How to approach gluten in your diet?

ACTION STEPS

1. Try a gluten-free diet for 3-6 months and keep a strict log of your symptoms (monitor pain, swelling, and stiffness in your joints every 2-3 weeks). Use my Rheumatoid Arthritis Journal listed in the resource section for an easy logging method (available on amazon.com).
2. Incorporate more gluten-free whole grains (quinoa, wild rice, corn) in your diet.
3. Replace white bread with gluten-free whole-grain bread.
4. Replace white pasta with gluten-free whole-grain pasta.

Nightshade Vegetables

Lucy was 45 years old when she stepped into my clinic complaining of pain, stiffness, and mild swelling around her knuckles and thumbs. During our appointment, she shared

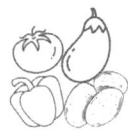

with me that her stiffness was worse in the morning but seemed to improve as the day went on.

When I asked her how long she'd been experiencing these symptoms, Lucy paused, saying, "I think around harvest time." Lucy loved to garden, and when her symptoms began, she'd thought she'd just been working too hard harvesting her home-grown vegetables.

As I heard her story, I grew concerned that she might have inflammatory arthritis. I ordered some tests, and when they came back, I noticed only a slight increase in her inflammation marker values and the rheumatoid factor (see Chapter 3 for more details about the RA diagnosis). I ordered X-rays of both of her hands, which was normal.

When Lucy came back for her follow-up, I told her that she likely suffered from a mild form of RA. Her face wrinkled, and I could see she'd begun to sweat just a little. She choked up and explained that throughout her life, she'd tried to live healthy. She wasn't ready to accept a lifelong disease.

When I suggested she try a mild medication to decrease some of her inflammation, Lucy asked, "Could I try and manage it through diet first?"

I smiled at her, saying, "Absolutely! Let's find out if there are any food triggers in your diet." I asked Lucy to keep a food diary and to return in 2 weeks. When she came back, I noticed that Lucy was a tomato-lover. She ate them daily—in soups, salads, stews, you name it!

When I asked her about this, she said, "My tomatoes did well this year, and I don't want to waste them—is that bad?"

"No, it's not bad, but some people are sensitive to tomatoes—they contain a substance called solanine that can cause inflammation in the gut, which causes inflammation in the body, including your joints! How about laying them off for a few months?"

Lucy agreed, ready to try anything to get some relief. She took a break from her favorite food and waited to see if her symptoms subsided. Three months later, she returned for a follow-up: Not only had her symptoms disappeared, but her follow-up tests were back to normal.

Tomatoes are a type of nightshade vegetable, along with eggplants, white potatoes, and a few others. As I told Lucy, nightshade vegetables are a part of the Solanaceae plant family, and solanine, the substance in these vegetables, is an alkaloid compound known to cause gut inflammation and leaky gut, both of which are causes for concern for RA patients.

What are the nightshade vegetables?

- White potatoes
- Tomatoes
- Eggplant
- Bell peppers
- Cayenne pepper
- Paprika

While I usually encourage patients to consume a diet rich in plant-based foods, nightshade vegetables are an exception. Studies link frequent consumption of white potatoes and tomatoes with gut inflammation, leaky gut, and a higher risk of developing inflammatory bowel diseases (IBS).[18] Like Lucy, many RA patients report more inflammation, stiffness, and pain after eating these vegetables.

While not everyone is sensitive to nightshade vegetables, I still suggest replacing these with another type of vegetable with anti-inflammatory properties (see the table below for a complete list).

Nightshade vegetables	Replace with...
White potatoes Eggplants Tomatoes Bellpeppers Cayenne pepper	Cauliflower Sweet potatoes Mushrooms Carrots Beets Zucchini Celery Pumpkin Onion Garlic

Coffee

Who doesn't enjoy a warm cup of coffee in the morning? I certainly do! 400 million cups of coffee are consumed daily in the U.S. alone, and coffee consistently ranks among our favorite beverages worldwide.[19] While coffee remains among the world's most widely consumed beverages, the jury is out on whether or not coffee causes and exacerbates RA.

A systemic analysis of over 250,000 participants found that those consuming caffeinated coffee were at 6% higher risk for RA.[20] Additionally, those who drank decaffeinated coffee were at 11% higher risk for developing RA. Scientists believe that some of the chemicals in coffee exert a pro-inflammatory response, causing higher levels of inflammation markers that prime the body for the disease. However, other studies found no significant association between coffee consumption and RA, so the evidence remains murky.[21]

Based on these results and the evidence I've collected anecdotally, I don't believe caffeine is the problem with coffee. Instead, cream and sugar, commonly added to caffeinated and decaffeinated coffee, cause inflammation in the body.

> Does coffee impact RA Treatment? Some studies looking specifically at patients treated with methotrexate found that drinking coffee decreased the treatment's efficacy, but others didn't confirm these findings. [22,23]

I urge my patients to consider replacing coffee with green tea: The same study that found that coffee contributes to RA found that those who drank more than three cups of green tea daily were at a decreased risk of developing RA (we'll discuss green tea in more depth in later sections).

In previous sections, we discussed sugar's role in inflammation, and I believe it's genuinely the culprit causing uncomfortable and unnecessary inflammation in coffee-drinking RA patients. Drink coffee in moderation, but avoid adding extra sugar and cream to help reduce inflammation and pain. Better yet, consider replacing coffee with green tea.

After Elimination: What's Next?

You've gotten rid of the debris and toxins stopping you from taking charge of your body: You've cut out excess sugar and salt, traded gluten-heavy foods for whole grains, limited your saturated and trans fat intake, and you've stopped consuming too many tomatoes and potatoes. Habits are difficult to break, and elimination is the hardest step for many of my patients. Feel free to celebrate—you're finally taking the first step to cleaning up your diet and taking charge of your symptoms!

Healing Your Body 101

What's next? And, more importantly, what's possible? Now, it's time for more of the good stuff!

Think back to the cleaning metaphor at the beginning of the chapter: Like certain cleaning products that 'go' with specific tasks and surfaces, certain foods are good for your RA. In this section, we'll talk about how to heal your gut to heal your body. We'll introduce how, and most importantly, why it's essential to heal your gut by introducing lots of fibers from whole grains, colorful fruits, and vegetables, and we will discuss the role of probiotics and prebiotics. Plus, I will teach you why spicing up your plate with cumin, ginger, or garlic helps decrease the inflammation in your body. We will finish the chapter by introducing you to RA-friendly diets. We'll also discuss what, how, and why—you deserve to know the facts.

It's not just about what you don't eat—it's about what you eat. These foods are scientifically proven to benefit RA patients, relieving inflammation and less pain and fatigue. Instead of reaching for what you think is healthy, go for any of these scientifically proven beneficial foods for your RA.

It's a lifestyle, not a diet. And because no diet is sustainable, your lifestyle will shape your healthy future and allow you to use as little prescription medicine as possible.

It's time to supercharge your diet—let's get started!

Healing Your Gut with More Fiber

Healing your body starts with healing your gut. In Chapter 4, we've covered a lot about the connection between our microbiome and the immune system and the importance of these two living in harmony. This is particularly important in patients with RA, where changing what they eat will affect their gut microbiome.

Throughout this book, we've briefly touched on fiber's role in regulating, modulating, and healing your gut and, therefore, your painful inflammation. In this section, we'll discuss the importance of not only eating more fiber but also how it aids in healing your gut microbiome.

> **○ PROTIP**
> Fiber is readily found in fruits, vegetables, and legumes, in addition to whole grains.

What *is* fiber? Fiber is a complex carbohydrate that can't be broken down like 'normal' carbohydrates, like sucrose. Instead, fiber passes right through the colon.

There are two types of dietary fiber: soluble and insoluble. Many plant 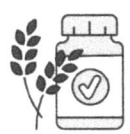 foods contain both types of fibers in different proportions. For example, plants are typically high in insoluble fibers comprising the cell walls. Insoluble fiber doesn't dissolve in water or gastrointestinal fluids, passing through the colon unaltered. During its journey, insoluble fibers 'stick' to other byproducts of the body's digestive system, preventing constipation and easing food's passage through the bowel. While beneficial, these fibers can't be fermented by the gut microbiome but play an essential role in absorbing excess fluid.

Soluble fibers, on the other hand, dissolve in both water and gastrointestinal fluids, forming a gel-like substance fermented by the colon's bacteria and releasing a few calories. Soluble fibers are critical—they serve as food for your gut microbiome. Scientists call these MAC fibers, or microbiome-accessible carbohydrates because they feed the gut microbiome and keep it happy and healthy. But that's not all. MAC fiber fertilizes MAC fibers, which produce short-chain fatty acids, or SCFAs.

> *Soluble fibers are critical—they serve food for your gut microbiome and maintain our diversity of gut species. Fermentation of soluble fibers leads to short-chain fatty acids.*

Why do we need fiber? There are many reasons, but perhaps most importantly, fiber is critical to maintaining gut species diversity. Through his research, Dr. Knight, creator of the American Gut Project, found that eating at least 30 different plants per week is the highest predictor of gut diversity and that people eating various plant foods had more SCFA-producing bacteria. His research illustrates a key takeaway: The more plants we eat, the healthier our bacteria are, and, by proxy, the better we feel.

What are the benefits of fiber for your health?

- Decrease inflammation and reduce the risk of developing autoimmune disease
- Prolong the absorption of dietary cholesterol, decreasing the risk of heart disease
- Keep you fuller for longer periods, reducing the risk of obesity
- Prolong the absorption of glucose in the gut, lowering the risk of diabetes
- Prevent constipation and hemorrhoids

The More Fiber, the More SCFAs

SCFAs aren't to be overlooked. They're communicators responsible for mediating messages between your gut microbiome and your immune system. Imagine them like negotiators, taking information from one, and sending it to the other. Furthermore, the more SCFAs you have, the more healthy gut bacteria you have: More of one boosts the other.

Beyond communication, SCFAs wear many hats. They are the primary energy source for colon cells, and they are fed, too. Secondly, SCFAs also make the colon more acidic, preventing the growth of inflammatory and pathogenic bacteria such as salmonella and E. Coli, restoring dysbiosis, and balancing good and bad bacteria in the gut. Lastly, SCFAs help repair leaky gut syndrome, preventing the absorption of harmful bacteria and toxins and lessening inflammation. Thus, SCFAs play an important, if not vital, role in our health.

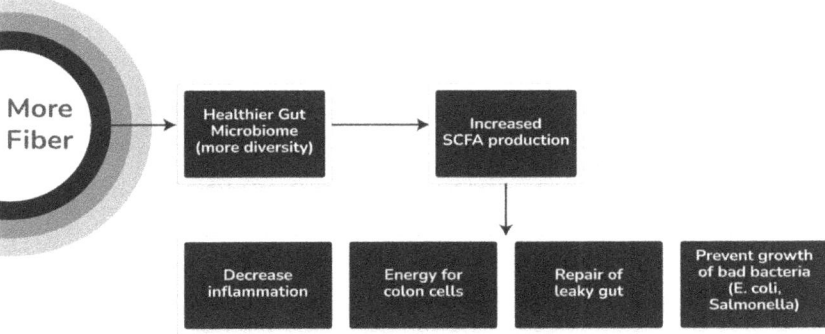

Figure 2. Effects of a High-Fiber Diet on the Microbiome

Whole-grains rich in fiber
- Oats
- Barley
- Wheat
- Bulgur
- Rye
- Quinoa
- Brown rice

But why is this important for RA patients or those struggling with inflammation? Here's the gist: Fiber generates SCFAs, and SCFAs help us fight inflammation. Studies show that those who consume more soluble fibers generate more SCFA, and the more SCFAs we have, the lower our inflammation levels.[24] For example, people adopting a Mediterranean or vegetarian diet—both high in fiber—have higher SCFA levels and fewer pro-inflammatory molecules in their bodies.[25] Plus, more SCFA helps you feel less fuller for longer, reducing blood glucose levels and helping you lose weight, which can be a decisive factor in the RA healing process.

Without Fiber, What Happens?

When gut bacteria don't have access to dietary fiber, they find another easily accessible carbohydrate source—the intestinal mucus lining. Thus, the gut bacteria feast on mucus and slowly but surely compromise the mucosal lining, the barrier between your intestines and your body's inside world. This process signals your immune system cells lined up under the intestinal mucosa, resulting in inflammation.

> ○ **PROTIP**
>
> **The American Heart Association recommends a daily dietary fiber intake of 25 to 30 grams from food, not fiber supplements.**

This is a significant problem, considering that most Americans eat less than the minimum fiber needed to supply the rest of their health needs (including SCFA production). In 1977, the Food and Drugs Administration recommended that Americans increase their fiber consumption; 38 grams is recommended daily for men, and 29 grams is recommended daily for women. Unfortunately, only 5% of Americans meet or exceed these guidelines, with 95% consuming only 15 grams of fiber daily—not even half of what is recommended.[26]

In 2019, a study on RA patients found that those who gradually increased their fiber consumption from 15 to 30 g a day showed a greater number of circulating regulatory T-cells, which are responsible for regulating the body's inflammatory response.[27] This response translates to less visible inflammation and, in the study, fewer swollen and eroded joints. Furthermore, all of these benefits improve patients' pain.

Where can you get fiber?

Now that I've explained the importance of fiber in healing your gut, we come to another frequently asked question: Where do we get more fiber? Throughout the next section of this chapter, I will introduce you to foods high in fiber, including whole grains, fruits, vegetables, legumes, and healthy nuts and seeds.

Increase your fiber consumption gradually. Each week, bump up the amount you eat to avoid abdominal discomfort. Aim for 25-30 grams of fiber daily from food sources, and check out the meal plan below to get started.

> ○ **PROTIP**
>
> Remember to drink 2.5-3 liters of water (100 fl oz) when increasing fiber intake to ensure smooth digestion.

Whole Grains

As we touched on in the elimination section, not all gluten, grains, bread, and wheat products are 'bad' for you! Some grain products, like whole grains, are healthy, proven to help digestion and to lessen inflammation.

Whole grains contain all three parts of the original grain (they're a plant, after all), including the bran, germ, and endosperm. The bran is the outer layer of the kernel, containing plenty of fiber, B vitamins, minerals, and antioxidants. The bran is also rich in phytochemicals, naturally derived plant compounds that prevent disease and contribute to overall health. Fiber in the bran slows the breakdown of the starch you consume into glucose, maintaining healthy blood sugar levels instead of the spikes you experience when you eat foods rich in simple sugars. Next is the germ: Rich in vitamins E and B, phytochemicals, and antioxidants, as well as healthy fats, the germ is the core where the seed grows. Lastly, the endosperm is the kernel's outer layer. The endosperm is rich in carbohydrates and protein but contains fewer nutrients than other parts of the whole grain kernel.

Hundreds of years ago, all grains were whole. However, modern processing techniques bleach flour and remove the germ and bran, leaving only the endosperm. This process is designed to boost flour's self-life and appearance, but it renders much of it innutritious, as most of wheat's nutrients and fiber reside in the germ and bran. Unfortunately, most breads, cereals, crackers, desserts, and pastries are made with refined grains or ultra-processed flour, meaning what's left is starchy and nutrient-poor.

When you go to the grocery store, choose whole grain products. These are high in fiber that feeds and rebalances your gut microbiome and helps fight your pesky RA symptoms.

> ○ **PROTIP**
>
> When you see "whole grain" advertised on the food you buy, look at the list of ingredients and ensure that 'whole grains' appear first, or close to first, on the list.

How to increase your intake of whole grains?

ACTION STEPS

1. Swap your typical "grain" products for whole grains. For example, trade regular pasta for whole-grain pasta, and white bread should be traded for whole-grain bread.
2. Once a week, cook a meal with brown rice.
3. Check ingredient lists for 'whole' or 'whole grain. And ensure they appear first on the list of ingredients.

Fruits

Fruits contain high levels of phytochemicals that yield an anti-inflammatory effect on the body and joints. Studies show that phytochemicals exhibit an anti-inflammatory mechanism that lessens inflammation. Furthermore, eating fruits high in phytochemicals (such as flavonoids, carotenoids, etc.) can modulate gene expression and impact how you feel living with certain diseases like RA.

For RA patients specifically, fruits are a superfood: Studies show those who consume more fruit, berries in particular, are less likely to experience inflammation, joint pain, and morning stiffness than those who don't.[29] For example, in 2017, researchers gave arthritis patients a daily drink of freeze-dried strawberries for 12 weeks.[30] After the study, participants reported a significant improvement in their quality of life, inflammation, and pain levels, highlighting fruit's influential role in lessening inflammation and pain. A similar study on blueberries found that RA patients who consumed one cup of blueberries with a daily meal enjoyed significantly lowered markers of inflammation.[31]

○ **PROTIP**

Eating more berries, blueberries, strawberries, and pomegranates is recommended for patients with RA. Eating more berries, blueberries, strawberries and pomegranates are recommended in patients with RA.

Pomegranate is also an exceptional fruit to consider in your nutrition plan. It is also high in fiber, antioxidants, vitamins C and K, folate, potassium, and copper. Pomegranates have been shown to reduce oxidative stress on your body on the cellular level, preventing excessive inflammation for those suffering from RA.[32] Packing a two-fold punch, pomegranate consumption can even reduce your risk of developing cancer and diabetes.

Additionally, fruits are abundant in flavonoids, vitamins, and minerals and are a great source of fiber that will feed and heal your gut microbiome, another common concern for RA patients.

Therefore, eating more fruit, including berries such as blueberries, strawberries, and pomegranates, can help soothe and mitigate pain and inflammation.

○ PROTIP

The darker or more vibrant the color of a given fruit, the healthier and more beneficial it will be! Think about berries and blackberries.

Blueberry Blast Smoothie

Ingredients:

1 cup frozen or fresh blueberries (or replace with strawberries or raspberries)

1 frozen banana

1 cup Greek plain yogurt

1 cup fresh spinach

1/2 teaspoon vanilla extract

A few drops of lemon juice

1/2 cup almond milk

1/2 tablespoon almond butter

Instructions:

1. Combine all ingredients in a blender.
2. Blend on high speed until smooth and creamy, about 1-2 minutes. You may add more almond milk to thin the smoothie.
3. Pour into glasses and enjoy your nutritious and delicious Blueberry Blast Smoothie!

Prep Time: 5 minutes

Servings: 2

Beyond your garden-variety fruits and berries, enzymatic fruits, such as mango, papaya, and pineapple, yield promising benefits for RA patients. Enzymatic fruits naturally contain enzymes that help your digestive system break down large protein molecules. Without these enzyme's assistance, the gut can't break down large proteins, causing bloating, abdominal pain, and a lot of uncomfortable gas. Left unchecked, these proteins can cause inflammation, causing more pain.

> ○ **PROTIP**
>
> Pineapple contains the enzyme bromelain, papaya contains papain, and mangoes are high in amylases. These natural enzymes help ferment large proteins, which would otherwise increase inflammation.

Enzymatic fruits are powerful foods, especially for those struggling with RA. For example, bromelain in bananas is a powerful and long-used treatment for many inflammatory diseases; bromelain can regulate and modulate your body's immune system response, lessening it or fine-tuning it accordingly.[33] Papin, an enzyme in papayas, also yields anti-inflammatory properties on the body, though this one has been studied less.[34]

Golden Boost Smoothie

Ingredients:

1/2 cup (80g) frozen cubed mango

1 fresh banana

1/2 cup (105g) cubed pineapple

½ cup plain Greek yogurt

1 cup (240ml) unsweetened almond milk

1 tablespoon of ground flaxseed

1/2 teaspoon of turmeric powder

Mint leaves for garnish

Instructions:

1. Add all the ingredients to a blender.
2. Blend on high speed until smooth and creamy, about 1-2 minutes. You may add more almond milk to thin the smoothie.
3. Pour into glasses and enjoy your nutritious and delicious
4. Mint leaves on top to garnish

Prep Time: 5 minutes
Servings: 2

Many so-called "nutrition gurus" on social media will warn you about excess fructose in fruits. Still, there is no indication eating fruit is linked to liver disease or other conditions typically associated with fructose consumption. If you have diabetes, adjust the amount of fruits you consume—don't leave them out entirely.

Because of their vast benefits, I encourage patients to include all types of fruit in their daily nutrition plans. Eat fruits of all colors, from pineapple, mango, and papaya to berries, cherries, pomegranates, grapes, and apples. Food is medicine, so I encourage my patients to incorporate fruit into their diet as a potent anti-inflammatory tool.[35]

> **How to increase your intake of fruits?**
> ACTION STEPS
> 1. Consume a colorful plate of fruits: Aim to eat a rainbow of fruits each week.
> 2. Eat all the fruits available in the season
> 3. If you have this option, aim to eat pineapple, mango, or papaya twice or thrice weekly.
> 4. Fresh vs frozen fruits. Both are acceptable options, especially when fruits are out of season.
> 5. Use smoothies as an easy way to incorporate fruits into your diet.

Green Vegetables

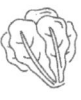

High in vitamins A, K, C, and E and fiber, green vegetables are widely understood to pack a strong nutrient punch. Common examples of green vegetables include:

Leafy Greens	Non-Leafy Greens
Spinach	Asparagus
Kale	Broccoli
Swiss chard	Brussels sprouts
Collard greens	Cucumbers
Arugula	Green beans
Romaine lettuce	Green bell peppers
Bok choy	Okra
Watercress	Peas
Mustard greens	Zucchini
Beet greens	

Each of these vitamins yields its own benefits: Vitamin E is a powerful antioxidant that boosts the immune system and lowers the risk of developing heart disease. Vitamin K in spinach and kale decreases inflammation and free radical production, healing the body's cells. Furthermore, a 2022 study on more than 30,000 participants from Korea showed that doubling a patient's vitamin B1, B2, and omega-3 fatty acids decreased their risk of developing RA, osteoarthritis, and heart disease.[36]

> Leafy green vegetables are the basis of both the vegetarian and the Mediterranean diets, which yield fantastic benefits for RA patients.

Leafy greens are rich in these vitamins, hence their importance in your RA-symptom-busting nutrition plan!

How to increase your intake of green vegetables?

ACTION STEPS

1. If you aren't used to green vegetables, especially leafy greens, gradually incorporate them into your meal plan. Start with twice a week and aim to get to 6 times per week.
2. Try adding green vegetables to your smoothies or omelets. Eat them baked, steamed, or in a salad.]

Green Juice Recipe

Ingredients:

1 cup spinach

1 peeled cucumber

1 peeled kiwi

1/2 lime, skin cut off

1/2 teaspoon fresh ginger

1 teaspoon freshly chopped parsley

1/2 glass of sparkling water

Instructions:

1. Wash and chop the spinach, cucumber, kiwi, lime, and ginger.
2. Put everything through the juicer.
3. Dilute with water if it's too thick.
4. Enjoy immediately!

Prep Time: 5 minutes

Servings: 2

Broccoli and Avocado Salad

Ingredients:

2 cups (180g) broccoli, cut into florets

1 avocado, pitted and chopped

3 eggs, hard-boiled (or replace with tofu for a vegetarian option)

For the dressing:

2 tablespoons plain Greek yogurt

1 teaspoon of olive oil

1 teaspoon of fresh lemon juice

1 teaspoon of freshly chopped parsley

Pinch of salt and pepper

Instructions:

1. Boil salted water in a small pot and cook broccoli for about 3-5 minutes, until tender.
2. Mix all the ingredients for the dressing in a small bowl.
3. Place the cooked broccoli, chopped avocado, and hard-boiled eggs (or tofu) in a bowl.
4. Drizzle with the dressing and season with salt and pepper.
5. Toss gently to combine, then serve and enjoy!

Substitution: Replace broccoli with cauliflower for a different twist.

Prep Time: 10 minutes

Cook Time: 5 minutes

Servings: 2

Legumes

Legumes are a type of plant from the Fabaceae family. The term 'legume' refers to the entire plant, including the leaves, stems, and pods. The seeds of these plants are the 'beans' and come in the form of peas, seeds, beans, or lentils.

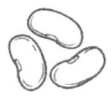

High in critical nutrients such as fiber, B-complex vitamins (including B1, B2, and B6), and vital minerals including iron, calcium, potassium, phosphorous, and zinc, legumes have a low glycemic index, meaning they help your body control its glucose levels, lowering the risk of diabetes. Furthermore, legumes aid with satiety, helping you feel fuller, which can aid in weight loss.

Legumes to incorporate into your meals
- Beans (different species)
- Peas
- Edamame
- Garbanzo beans
- Lentils
- Soy nuts
- Peanuts

○ **PROTIP**

Lentils and beans are fantastic healthy protein substitutes. People on a vegetarian or vegan diet consume these high amounts to ensure adequate protein intake.

What about those with RA? Firstly, legumes are high in fiber, increasing SCFA production and less inflammation. One study looked at legumes and their effect on inflammation markers for six weeks and found that participants charged with consuming more legumes showed fewer markers of inflammation than the group who didn't.[37] Other studies indicate that eating these mighty beans can help fight inflammation.[38]

As discussed in the last section, fiber's role in fighting inflammation is a powerful component of any RA patient's meal plan. Legumes are exceptionally high in this critical nutrient group, so I highly recommend all my patients use them to combat their symptoms.

How to incorporate more legumes into your meals?

ACTION STEPS

1. Try different legumes (beans, lentils, chickpeas, etc). Aim at least three times/ week.
2. Before you cook the beans or lentils, let them soak for about 12-24 hours, as this practice improves their nutrient content and helps them become more easily digested.

Creamy Lentil and Vegetable Soup

Ingredients:

1 tablespoon of olive oil

1 white or sweet onion, peeled and diced

1 medium carrot, diced

1 celery stalk, diced

2 cloves of garlic, minced

4 cups of vegetable stock

1 cup of red lentils, rinsed and soaked for a few hours

1/2 teaspoon of ground cumin

1/2 teaspoon of curry powder (optional)

Pinch of saffron

Zest and juice of 1/2 lemon

Salt and pepper, to taste

Instructions:

1. Rinse lentils and soak in water for a few hours before cooking.
2. Heat oil in a large stockpot over medium-high heat. Add onion, carrots, celery, and sauté for five minutes, stirring occasionally, until the onions are soft and translucent.
3. Add garlic and sauté for one more minute, stirring occasionally, until fragrant.
4. Stir in the vegetable stock, lentils, cumin, and curry powder (plus saffron, if using) until combined. Continue cooking until the soup reaches a simmer. Then cover and cook for 20-30 minutes, stirring occasionally, until the lentils are completely tender.
5. Using either a hand or traditional blender, puree the soup until it reaches your desired consistency.
6. Season with salt and pepper. Stir in the lemon zest and juice until combined.
7. Serve warm.

Prep Time: 10 minutes

Cook Time: 30 minutes

Serving: 2

Nuts and Seeds

Nuts are a fantastic source of fiber (see earlier in the chapter for more details), vitamin E, and micronutrients, including selenium, magnesium, and copper. They're also loaded with powerful antioxidants, which reduce stress on your body's cells and fight inflammation. Furthermore, nuts yield impressive effects on cholesterol and triglyceride levels, which are known to contribute to heart disease, diabetes, and obesity, which often exist concurrently with RA.

The first study illustrating the benefits of eating nuts came from one examining the Mediterranean diet: Participants were separated into three groups, one who ate a Mediterranean diet (more on this to come), one group who ate a Mediterranean diet supplemented with thirty grams of nuts, and a control group.[39] The 'nutty group,' as I call it, showed a 30% lowered risk of major cardiovascular events over five years, and a 45% lessened risk of stroke.

But what about inflammation? Another similar study showed that those who ate a Mediterranean diet supplemented with nuts experienced significantly less inflammation than those who didn't, indicating nuts' potential anti-inflammatory properties.[40] Additionally, compared to their counterparts, these participants enjoyed lowered C-reactive protein and interleukin-6 (both proteins that create inflammation in the body).

Different types of nuts
- Walnuts
- Cashew
- Pecans
- Pistachios
- Almonds
- Hazelnuts

Though nuts are relatively high in fats, the fats in nuts are called monounsaturated fats; these are the 'good' ones, and we'll discuss these in more depth later in the chapter. Unlike unhealthy saturated and trans fats, these contain healthy oils that maintain cognitive function and cell structure. However, remember that nuts are relatively energy-dense, meaning they're high in calories. Thirty grams is the recommended dose for adults—aim to eat just one handful a day.

> **Did you know that nuts can lower your lipid levels?**
> - Pistachios have been shown to lower triglycerides in those suffering from both obesity and diabetes.
> - Almonds and hazelnuts can raise 'good' HDL cholesterol while reducing total and 'bad' LDL cholesterol.

Nuts aren't the only small snack beneficial to your RA symptoms—seeds, including chia seeds and flax seeds, are highly nutritious sources of monounsaturated fats. Each is a great source of protein, antioxidants, and minerals which play a role in reducing cholesterol and your risk of heart disease.

Let's talk about seeds! Commonly available at your local grocery store, flaxseeds are the richest plant-based sources of alpha-linolenic acid (ALA), omega-3 fatty acid.

> **○ PROTIP**
>
> Use crushed or ground flaxseeds; this process makes it easier for your body to digest them.

Chia seeds, too, are an excellent source of ALA, but they pack their most significant punch in the form of fiber—just one serving of chia seeds yields about ten grams of fiber, which fills you up, maintains a healthy gut microbiome, and helps control weight and inflammation. Additionally, chia seeds can absorb liquid easily—when they do, they take on a jelly-like consistency conducive to certain puddings and oat recipes.

Both are high in necessary fiber, nuts, and seeds, and they yield powerful anti-inflammatory benefits on your body, helping you fight your RA symptoms from the inside out! Nuts and seeds are among my favorite afternoon snacks; I believe everyone (unless you're allergic) should include these in their RA symptom-busting plan.

Chia Seed Pudding with Mixed Berries

Ingredients:

1/4 cup of chia seeds

1 cup of almond/ oat milk

1 tablespoon of honey (optional)

1/2 teaspoon of vanilla extract

Mixed berries for topping (strawberries, blueberries, and raspberries)

Instructions:

1. Mix chia seeds, almond milk, and vanilla extract in a bowl.
2. Stir well to combine and let it sit for 5 minutes.
3. Stir the mixture again to break up any clumps of chia seeds.
4. Cover and refrigerate overnight, or for at least 2 hours, until the pudding has thickened.
5. Before serving, top the chia seed pudding with mixed berries.
6. Enjoy your delicious and nutritious chia seed pudding!

Prep Time: 5 minutes

Chilling Time: 2 hours or overnight

Serving: 1

How to incorporate more nuts and seeds?

ACTION STEPS

1. Eat nuts raw, or very lightly salted. You can place them in a preheated oven for just a few minutes or add them to your salads or smoothies.
2. Stir grounded flax seeds into yogurt with fruit. Try adding them to smoothies, cereal, or on a salad.
3. Add chia seeds to smoothies and oatmeal—remember, they absorb liquid easily!

Probiotics

Probiotics are tiny, living organisms that boost the number of good bacteria 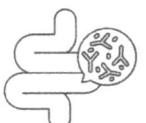 in your gut. The supplement market advertises probiotics as a cure for all problems, but this isn't quite the case. Let's discuss here how probiotics will impact people with RA.

I liken probiotics to 'gut tourists.' They're transient members of your gut microbiome, passing into the gut as you take them (or consume probiotic-heavy foods) and leaving with regular excretion. Hence, consuming them regularly is essential to maintain their health benefits.

Research shows that RA patients benefit from probiotics, particularly while following their treatment plan. A meta-analysis showed that people with RA who used a probiotic had lower inflammation markers, illustrating the probiotic's potential role in lessening inflammation.[41] Another study of sixty women with RA used the lactobacillus casei bacterium, a probiotic, for eight weeks.[42] At the end of the study, those using the probiotic had lower levels of inflammation, fewer swollen and tender joints, and lowered overall disease activity. Better yet—they had no side effects.

> ○ **PROTIP**
>
> Look for foods fermented in salted water rather than vinegar, as chemicals in vinegar will kill all living bacteria.

We'll discuss probiotic supplements in Chapter 6, but for now, let's discuss their place on the table—in the foods you regularly consume. Fermented foods are rich in probiotics and help you maintain gut microbiome diversity. Check out the bullets for a few examples.

- Yogurt
- Cultured sour cream
- Sauerkraut
- Pickles
- Kombucha
- Kefir
- Kimchi
- Fermented grains and fish

These foods are rich in probiotics, which help heal your gut microbiome, improve inflammation, and generate more SCFA. Aim to eat more of these foods to keep your RA at bay.

> **How to increase the probiotic foods intake?**
> ACTION STEPS
> 1. Gradually introduce fermented foods into your nutrition plan.
> 2. Start your day with yogurt or kefir.
> 3. Introduce pickles and sauerkraut, both fermented foods, into your diet. Consume them weekly.

Prebiotics

The word 'prebiotic' sounds a little like 'probiotic,' but the two are far from the same: Unlike probiotics, *prebiotics aren't living organisms*. Rather, prebiotics are 'food' for your gut bacterium; ingesting them increases the number of good bacteria living in your colon.

Available as both a supplement and in the foods we eat, prebiotics are a form of complex carbohydrate (long chains of linked sugar molecules) that can't be absorbed or metabolized by the gut. Like fiber, they feed and are fermented by the microbiome, promoting good bacteria growth, abundance, and diversity.

Inulin is among the most common forms of probiotics. It's a polymer of up to sixty fructose molecules (a sugar molecule) linked together, commonly found in fruits and vegetables. The body can't break down inulin, but when it reaches the colon, gut bacteria can break the bonds between inulin's fructose molecules, releasing sugar and, thus, food. Gut bacteria ferment inulin, producing SCFA and protecting the gut from inflammation. Animal studies of inulin and RA specifically show that inulin and a probiotic can reduce and lessen RA symptoms.[43]

Which foods naturally contain inulin?
• Chicory roots
• Dandelion greens
• Jerusalem artichoke
• Garlic
• Onions
• Bananas
• Leeks
• Asparagus
• Apples
• Cocoa
• Crushed Flaxseeds
• Seaweed

In short, probiotics heal the gut microbiome, yielding anti-inflammatory benefits for you and your disease. For maximum gut microbiome-boosting impact, combine probiotic and prebiotic foods; this forms a symbiotic relationship that feeds and nourishes your gut, and will improve your RA symptoms and pain.

Healthy Fats

As we alluded to in the earlier sections of this chapter, not all fats are bad. Good fats are responsible for a few important bodily processes, including energy storage, nerve cell structure, and protecting your internal organs.

Unsaturated fats are the 'good' kind. Derived from plant oils and seeds, they are a crucial part of your RA nutrition plan. These fats are separated into two categories: monounsaturated fatty acids (MUFA) and polyunsaturated fatty acids (PUFA).

MUFA (monounsaturated fatty acids) fats are readily available in plant products, such as avocados and nuts. Olive oil is an excellent example of MUFAs—on its own, it's a bit of a superfood. Studies show that regularly consuming olive oil can lead to a 30% decrease in your risk of developing heart disease, among other ailments.[44] Components of olive oil, including oleic acid, have natural anti-inflammatory properties. I recommend using unfiltered, cold-pressed olive oil in all of your salads.

PUFA fats, or polyunsaturated fatty acids, such as omega-3 fatty acids and omega-6 fatty acids, are essential. The body can't produce them on its own, so we must consume them from another source.

Found in pumpkin seeds, soybeans, walnuts, algae, sardines, certain egg varieties, and olive oil, omega-3 fatty acids, such as EPA and DHA (eicosapentaenoic acid and docosahexaenoic acid), yield an anti-inflammatory response in the body: They influence the COX-2 enzyme, the same one blocked by NSAID (non-steroidal anti-inflammatory drugs) medications, reducing inflammation.

Because of their anti-inflammatory role, omega-3 fatty acids are crucial for those struggling with RA. For example, fish are high in omega-3 fatty acids, and studies show that consuming more fatty fish profoundly reduces inflammation (check out the next chapter for more information on fish oil and omega-3s).[45]

> ○ **PROTIP**
>
> The American Heart Association (AHA) recommends eating at least two portions of fish per week, particularly oily fish rich in omega-3 fatty acids.

Historically, scientists believed a proper diet contained an equal omega-3 to omega-6 FAs (or a 1:1 ratio). However, our modern Western diets have ruined this ratio: Many Americans consume omega-6 and omega-3s at a 6:1 or even a 20:1 ratio. This is a significant problem: Omega-6 fatty acids, commonly found in eggs, beef (grain and corn-fed), sunflower oil, and corn oil, don't yield the same health benefits as omega-3 fatty acids and aren't proven to fight inflammation or support heart health.

To summarize, not all fats are bad. We can't, and it is not recommended to cut out fat entirely: Unsaturated fats, particularly omega-3 fatty acids, decrease body inflammation, including the joint inflammation experienced by RA patients. Peruse the information in the later sections to learn about food sources of healthy fats.

Table 3. Seafood rich in Omega-3s PUFA

Seafood Variety		Content EPA+DHA mg/ 4oz
Omega-3 RICH PUFA Seafood	Salmon, Atlantic	1200-2400
	Anchovies, herring	2300-2400
	Mackerel, Atlantic and Pacific (not king)	1350-2100
	Tuna (Bluefin, Albacore)	1700
	Oysters Pacific	1550
	Sardines, Atlantic and Pacific	1100-1600
	Trout (freshwater)	1000-1100
	Tuna (albacore, canned)	1000
	Salmon (pink and sockeye)	700-900
	Swordfish	1000
	Shark	1250
Omega-3 POOR PUFA Seafood	Squid	750
	Crab: blue, king, snow, queen	200-550
	Tuna canned	150-300
	Clams	200-300
	Catfish	100-250
	Cod Atlantic and Pacific	200
	Scallops	200
	Lobsters	200
	Tilapia	150
	Mackerel king	450
	Shrimp	100

Note: This table was adapted from the American Heart Association [46]

Spice Up Your Food

Spices—and humans' use of them for health and food—have existed since ancient times. The practice of using spices to flavor food or medicinally spread through the Middle East, the Mediterranean, and parts of Asia. Over the past several decades, science has proved that many spices play an important role in preventing common diseases such as asthma, cancer, heart disease, diabetes, and RA.

Spices come from plants' roots, leaves, and seeds. Some are dried and ground up, while others, such as bay leaves, are sold whole for cooking.

Garlic, ginger, black pepper, cinnamon, basil, and turmeric are the most commonly used spices today.

In this section, we'll introduce these spices, specifically looking at each in the context of how—and most importantly, why—each is effective for treating your RA symptoms. For a more in-depth discussion of a few of these, feel free to check out Chapter 6 they can also be found in the form of supplements). Let's get started!

Turmeric

Often called 'the golden spice,' turmeric comes from the root of the *Curcuma longa* plant, native to southern Asia. Its active ingredient, curcumin, gives turmeric its yellow, golden color. This spice has been used in Asian dishes for centuries, but more recent studies revealing its antioxidant and anti-inflammatory properties have made it a common one in many kitchens around the world.[47]

Many studies illustrate curcumin's effectiveness at treating RA symptoms: Curcumin not only alleviates inflammation and pain but has been shown to modulate immune system cells, stopping the body's natural pain response.[47]

Because many don't often use turmeric in cooking, consider opting for a curcumin supplement to help fight inflammation. Check out the supplement chapter for a more in-depth discussion of curcumin and its benefits.

> ○ **PROTIP**
>
> Consume black pepper along with tumeric to boost its absorption.

Ginger

Today, ginger is more often used for culinary purposes than medicinal ones, but this doesn't mean it's any less beneficial for your health. From the same family as turmeric, ginger is used to treat nausea in pregnant women, but it also yields powerful antioxidant and anti-inflammatory benefits.

Studies show that RA patients consuming ginger, whether in supplement form or in food, report lowered disease activity, less discomfort, and less pain than those who don't.[48] Other studies found that ginger can be a powerful pain reliever, particularly for arthritis patients.[49]

Consider using ginger to alleviate some of your pain, and check out the supplement section for more information on ginger's scientifically-proven benefits.

Ginger has been scientifically proven to
- Lessen inflammation
- Lower inflammatory markers
- Lessen RA patients' reliance on medication
- Improve pain

Garlic

Garlic has long been used as a medication for longevity and as potential 'cure' 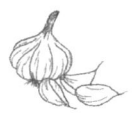 for heart disease. Today, few use garlic medicinally, and yet, its use in recipes still yields a variety of benefits. Garlic is both an antibacterial and anti-inflammatory, playing a critical role in preventing the development of certain chronic diseases.

Looking at RA more specifically, garlic's efficacy still stands: Human studies show that garlic interferes with inflammation, stopping its response.[50] Studies on RA patients show that those who consume garlic experience significantly less pain, fewer swollen joints, and less disease activity than those who don't.[51]

To glean these benefits, you may try it in supplement form or use more garlic in your food!

Pepper

Black and chili pepper are among the most commonly-used spices today, and each yield strong benefits for those with RA. Black pepper is widely known to yield antioxidant, anti-asthmatic, anti-carcinogenic, and unto-ulcerative properties. Chili pepper, used to provide a little extra kick to your plate, is often used as an analgesic (pain reliever and pain minimizer) in ointments, patches, and creams to help relieve patient's pain.

> **○ PROTIP**
>
> If you suffer from peripheral neuropathy, diabetic neuropathy, or post-herpetic neuropathy after shingles, use cream with capsaicin to ease your pain or discomfort.

Both chili pepper and black pepper aid in preventing and alleviating symptoms of many chronic conditions—RA included. Adding these spices to your diet yields cardiovascular benefits and their medicinal, anti-inflammatory, and anti-oxidative effects are widely understood to help alleviate RA symptoms.

> Per rheumatology guidelines, people with osteoarthritis (wear-and-tear arthritis) should try applying topical capsaicin to their joints as an alternative to other oral medication.

Combinations of these spices—garlic, turmeric, ginger, and peppers—yield solid benefits for your RA symptoms. Thus, a study that looked at the combination of ginger, garlic, cinnamon, and saffron (the latter two we didn't discuss, but you get the idea) was associated with boosted improvement to RA symptoms, with less pain and less swollen joints and can be an easy way to combat your pain naturally.[52] So, don't be afraid to mix and match when it comes to spices—replace your regular salt and sugar with these healthier options.

Green Tea

In the last section, we discussed the potential damage wrought on our systems by coffee, which has been shown to cause an inflammatory response (although it is still unclear if it is the coffee or the additions like creamers and sugar). However, the same study showed the beneficial effects of green tea.

Green tea contains polyphenols, a plant compound that provides anti-inflammatory and antioxidant benefits. In animal studies, green tea decreased the levels of pro-inflammatory cytokines and stopped the destruction of cartilage in the joints. In human studies, in elderly adults, who had been diagnosed with RA, green tea, when combined with exercise, lessened inflammation and other disease markers.[53] Interesting, right?

I often recommend to my RA patients that they trade their morning coffee for green tea. Green tea yields stark benefits for inflammation and pain and can help support weight loss, a common issue for many RA patients. Trade these as soon as possible to lessen your disease activity!

How to prepare green tea without the bitter taste?
- Add some water to your tea kettle, and let it boil.
- While it's boiling, prepare your tea bag or add tea leaves to a cup.
- Let the boiling water rest for 5 minutes.
- After this, let everything steep in the cup for three minutes, and remove it from the water.
- Now, enjoy!]

Supercharge 101 RA-friendly Diets

Now that you've cleaned the clutter from your diet and have things tidied up with healthier food options proven to alleviate pain and inflammation, it's time to supercharge!

In this section, I'll provide a few dietary frameworks to help you 'organize' and supercharge the way you think about food. As always, I'll tell you about the scientifically proven benefits of each. Understanding how, why, and what you can do to finally get back to feeling better and the more significant diets proven to help those suffering from RA provides the framework to do so. Let's get to supercharging!

The Mediterranean Diet

In the 1960s, scientists began noticing that people living in the Mediterranean region (parts of Greece and Italy) enjoyed fewer ailments such as heart disease, cognitive decline, and a longer lifespan. Further studies showed that these benefits were linked to the diet these people enjoyed, characterized by plants, few meat products, and whole foods. Today, recent studies confirmed that the Mediterranean is linked to

- Lower blood pressure, decrease heart disease risk
- Lower blood sugar and diabetes

- Decrease cholesterol levels
- Lower rates of cancers
- Lower rates of depression
- Less inflammation
- Longer lifespan

The foundation of the Mediterranean diet is the consumption—or abundance even—of whole foods. **Rather than a diet, it's a lifestyle:** The Mediterranean diet involves a more comprehensive look at your habits than other diets. Those following the Mediterranean diet shy away from the regimented exercise routines of those in Western countries; they opt to walk more and prioritize movement over stringently designed activities. One of my favorite hallmarks of this 'diet' is eating with friends and family and prioritizing eating at home. Those following this diet eat dinner with their family at set times and feel that food is a part of being in a community.

The Mediterranean diet is rather an eating pattern, not a diet. It is a lifestyle choice where cooking and enjoying food at home with family and friends, having social gatherings and walking to a store are a part of life, not a planned activity in your busy calendar.

On a more nutrient-focused level, the Mediterranean diet emphasizes whole, unprocessed foods above all else; those on this diet eat many plant-based foods, including fruits, vegetables, whole grains, nuts, and legumes (like beans), and enjoy dairy products, like yogurt and unprocessed cheese or eggs in moderation. Olive oil is a staple of the Mediterranean diet. The diet involves seasoning your foods with herbs and spices instead of excessive salt and sugar and cutting back on red meat, which is high in certain unhealthy fats. Instead, those following the diet consume plenty of fatty fish high in omega-3 fatty acids (including mackerel, herring, sardines, albacore tuna, and salmon). Added sugar isn't optimal in this diet, so cook most of your meals at home. Instead of unhealthy, baked desserts, those on this diet finish meals with yogurt, fresh fruit, and some honey. I'm not encouraging anyone to drink alcohol in excess. Still, studies have shown that those in Mediterranean countries who drink one glass of red wine (only one!) daily are healthier, as red wine is high in polyphenols and antioxidants.

Table 4. Mediterranean eating pattern

Type of Food	Goals for servings
Vegetables	≥ 2 servings/ day
Fresh Fruits	≥ 3 servings/ day (to be adjusted for diabetics)
Legumes	≥ 3 servings/ week
Fish	≥ 3 servings/ week
White Meat (poultry, turkey)	Instead of red meat
Olive Oil	≥ 4 tablespoons/day
Dairy Yogurt Milk	1 cup yogurt/day or 1 cup milk/ day (avoid if lactose-intolerant)
Nuts	≥ 3 servings/ week
Wine with meals	7 glasses/ week*
Soda drinks, commercially baked goods, pastries and sweets	< 1 drink/day <2 servings/week
Red and processed meats	< 1 servings/ day, better to avoid
Spread fats	< 1 servings/ day

Table adapted based on the information included in the PREDIMED Study 2018

So—does it work? Yes—it certainly does. One study of over 400 participants looked at the effects of a modified Mediterranean-type diet "that contained more bread, more root vegetables and green vegetables, more fish, fruit at least once daily, less red meat (replaced with poultry), and margarine with high content in alpha-linolenic acid [replaced] butter and cream."[54] After just under four years, study subjects who had followed the modified Mediterranean-type diet showed a 50-70% lower risk of heart disease, as well as a lower risk of stroke and pulmonary embolism. The study further found that the Mediterranean diet could potentially prevent cancer because it reduces oxidative damage, inflammation, and cell proliferation.

Looking at RA patients specifically, many promising scientific studies emerge: A recent (2018) study of over 1,700 patients with RA and nearly

4,000 control patients (those without RA) found that those who firmly adhered to a Mediterranean diet experienced a 21% decrease in their odds of developing RA.[55] Other studies show that those with RA when following a Mediterranean diet, enjoy fewer affected joints (swollen and painful joints), less pain, less inflammation, improved physical function, and overall lower disease activity than those who don't.

I highly recommend that all RA patients try the Mediterranean diet. Not only will it help control your inflammation, but this eating pattern and lifestyle will yield various health benefits, including less pain and improved physical functioning. Food is your body's fuel source—why not fuel it well?

Mediterranean diet best principles are summarized here

ACTION STEPS

1. Eat plenty of nuts and olives as a snack, or add them to your salads
2. Choose whole-grain products: bread or pasta.
3. Start each meal with a nice salad! Choose dark greens and top with seeds.
4. Make a habit of eating three legume servings / per week (beans, chickpeas, lentils, peas)
5. Replace more red meat with omega-3-rich fish, aiming to have at least three servings a week.
6. Replace sugar-beverages (e.g., soda, energy drinks) with water or green tea
7. Make a habit of eating fresh fruits for dessert
8. Eat your meals with your family and friends, and make dinner time a celebration of being together
9. If you can, walk to the grocery store instead of driving.

A Vegan Diet

You're likely already familiar with the vegan diet: Perhaps you have a friend or family member who consumes a largely vegetarian or vegan diet or a friend who avoids meat products. A *vegan* diet is entirely plant-based (there's that word again—I'm sensing a theme!), meaning that those following one consume a diet rich with plants, including vegetables and fruits, nuts, and grains. Unlike a *vegetarian* or *pescatarian* diet (those following these diets often consume dairy products like eggs and milk), those following a vegan diet don't consume any food product from an animal (animal byproducts included).[56] So, generally, vegans don't eat meat, dairy products, honey, or fish.

What foods *do* vegans eat?

- Tofu, tempeh, and seitan.
- Legumes
- Nuts and nut butter (peanut, almond, etc.)
- Seeds
- Plant-based milk (such as almond or oat milk)
- Nutritional yeast
- Algae
- Whole grains
- Vegetables and fruits (including fermented products)

Vegan diets provide many essential health benefits, including weight loss and maintenance due to their high consumption of plant-based fibers, which, as discussed earlier in the chapter, can aid in healing the gut microbiome. They also improve blood sugar levels, lower your risk of developing diabetes by up to 78%, and lower your risk of dying from heart disease by 42%.[57,58]

A recent 2023 study published in 2023 by Stanford researchers looked at the effect of implementing a vegan vs omnivorous, or 'traditional' diet in people who were twins to control many of the genetic differences that might alter the outcomes.[59] The vegan diet included vegetables, legumes, fruits, whole grains, nuts, and seeds. In just eight weeks, people who followed the vegan diet had significant benefits such as lower LDL cholesterol (the bad kind of cholesterol), lower fasting glucose, reduced body weight, and improved energy levels and overall well-being.

Looking at RA more specifically, a vegan diet has been shown to significantly improve your RA symptoms, including pain, swelling, and general inflammation. Based on a study in which people who were instructed to eat an uncooked vegan diet (participants consumed raw, plant based foods) experienced less pain and morning stiffness.[60] In addition, participants relied less on steroid medications and lower doses of methotrexate.

Health benefits of a vegan diet:
• Decreased diabetes risk
• Decreased cardiovascular risk
• Decreased blood pressure
• Lowers cancer risk
• Maintain normal weight
• Improves kidney function
• Lowers Alzheimer's disease risk

Why is this the case? A vegan diet more abundant in enzymatic fruits and fibrous foods helps the gut microbiome and decrease inflammation.

Other studies look more generally at the role of a vegan diet on RA; these studies report that RA patients following a vegan diet ate less fat, protein, and overall calories than their counterparts but increased their carbohydrate intake.[61] In this particular study, the patient's RA symptoms decreased significantly, and researchers noticed that inflammation marker levels were—generally—significantly reduced.

All of these findings show the importance and effectiveness of a vegan diet on your overall health and your RA symptoms. While some people may find this diet restricting, you may give it a try and track your symptoms.

The RA-Friendly Food Pyramid

This chapter covered a lot of information! If you found it overwhelming, you're not alone—much of this information can be difficult to digest (pun intended!). Luckily, I've collected and structured what I like to call the RA-Friendly Food Pyramid (inspired by an analysis of over 100 articles published about food and RA) to help RA patients decide what, why, and how often they should eat certain RA-friendly foods.[62] This food pyramid looks similar to the one you learned about in grade school, with a few key exceptions and caveats.

The lower part of the pyramid is those foods and habits you should regularly follow. At the bottom is regular, daily exercise, which we'll discuss

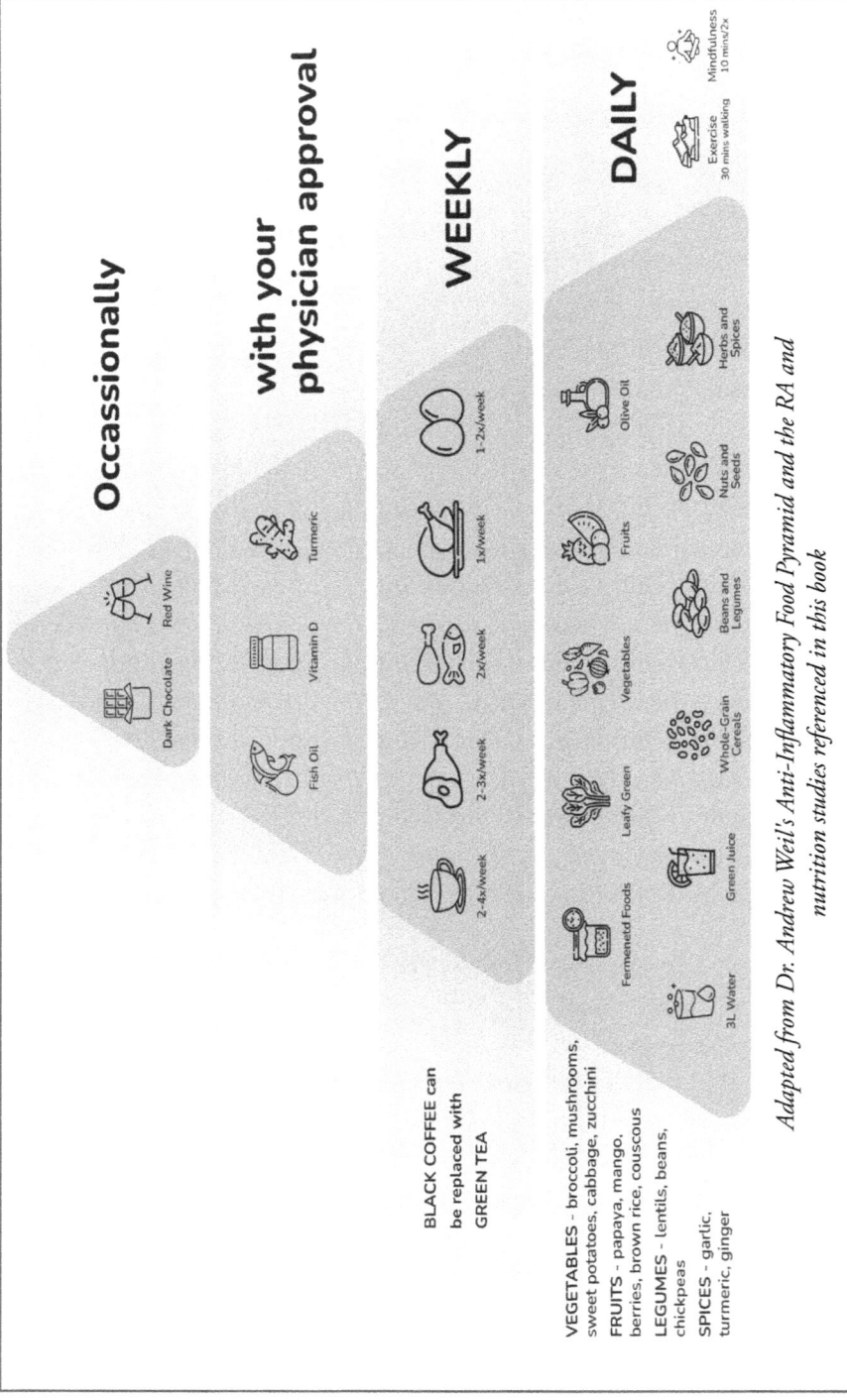

Adapted from Dr. Andrew Weil's Anti-Inflammatory Food Pyramid and the RA and nutrition studies referenced in this book in more depth in later sections. Water should also be the primary beverage of choice for RA patients. As we move upward, portions and days per week (which indicate the number of times you should consume the food shown) grow smaller. At the top, you can see that omega-3 fatty acids, vitamin D, and antioxidants are labeled in green and that salt and sugar (all of which we've previously discussed) are labeled in red as a warning.

This food pyramid is your 'key' to unlocking a pain-free future. RA is a lifelong diagnosis, and dietary and lifestyle interventions are meant to be followed as long as you have the disease. Therefore, it's important to follow them for the rest of your life, not just when your symptoms return.

RA requires lifelong dietary and lifestyle interventions, which must be adhered to consistently, not just during symptom flare-ups.

Reclaiming Your Future: Diet and RA

Finally—we've cleaned the house and, therefore, your diet! In the elimination section, we discussed all foods negatively impacting your RA, including salt and sugar, which aggravate inflammation; excessive saturated fats and vegetable oils, which negatively impact your gut microbiome; and, in certain people, the use of dairy and gluten.

Once we'd cleaned out the clutter, we moved on to healing, discussing which healthy ingredients you should add to your meal plan and the benefits of each. These foods, such as whole grains, fruits, leafy greens, vegetables, legumes, and spices heal your gut microbiome, decrease inflammation, and alleviate the pain you're experiencing.

Finally, in the last section, we moved onto supercharging, and discussed the more comprehensive meal plans you can use to 'reorganize' your food consumption. Use the Mediterranean, vegan, and RA-friendly diets to make larger, more sweeping changes to mitigate your symptoms.

Diet, particularly in the context of RA and other autoimmune diseases, is a key factor in alleviating painful symptoms. Without a focus on diet and without making these necessary—and likely overdue—changes, you risk joint damage, swelling, inflammation, and a stronger reliance on conventional medications.

Learn to see your RA differently: Your disease is a part of you, but your disease does not define you, nor does it have to consume your life. Treat your body as a whole entity–a mind, body, and soul—not just a collection of broken parts.

Now that we're finished cleaning up your space—your diet—it's time to move onward, upward, and into the other changes you can make to feel better.

Rheumatoid arthritis (RA) may be a part of your life, but it doesn't have to define you or consume your life. Treat your body as a whole—mind, body, and soul—not just a collection of broken parts.

CHAPTER 6

THE NOT-SO BITTER PILLS

Now that we've established your diet's vital role in how you feel living with RA, it's time to discuss a question that many of my patients ask me, "Can or should I take supplements for my RA?" And, a necessary follow-up, "Which ones should I take?"

Dietary supplements refer to vitamins, minerals, enzymes, herbs, botanicals, and amino acids taken in capsule, tablet, or gummy form. Many adults in the United States take supplements for various reasons, with Vitamins D and B12, omega-3s as well as daily multivitamins, being the most popular options.

When taken correctly, the right supplements can help RA patients boost their immune system, decrease inflammation, and lessen their reliance on medications (e.g., NSAIDs). Remember, however, that supplements won't replace your current medication regimen. They're an essential addition to your RA treatment but not a substitute.

Similar to the last chapter, I'll be introducing a lot of information, but this information is combined with action steps to help you quickly incorporate each of these steps into your life and take charge of your RA diagnosis! Let's begin!

Supplements 101

"Doctor G," Maria began. "I've been taking my meds, and I made some diet changes. I feel a little better, but I'm still in pain all the time." M years old when I diagnosed her with RA. However, after three years with this disease, she felt physically and emotionally drained. Maria was on three potent medications, including methotrexate, sulfasalazine, Plaquenil, and Celebrex twice daily, just like clockwork. Still, she complained of pain levels around 5/10.

"I've been reading up on supplements and even my friend recommended one with collagen and glucosamine, but I wanted to check with you. What do you suggest?" she asked me.

I knew that Maria wasn't interested in biologic medication, and we'd discussed that a few times. I wanted to respect her decision and said, "Maria, I appreciate your honesty and commitment to this." She nodded. "You know I'll always recommend something backed by science, right? Some studies show that certain supplements can help your treatment process. Some supplements can help—but not all that you see advertised. The supplements your friend recommended—glucosamine and collagen—aren't shown to be effective in RA patients."

Maria looked a little confused and replied, "Really? Is there another one I can try?"

"Yes, some studies show that fish oil benefits RA patients. Adding it to your medication regimen would be a good option."

"How much should I start with?" she asked.

"Start slow," I urged her. "Starting slowly will make sure you don't experience common side effects like an upset stomach. Begin with a gram a day for the first month, and if that goes well, we can increase your dosage to 2 grams daily."

Maria committed to this regimen and, during our follow-up three months later, she told me, "My pain's down to a 3/10!" After another six months, her pain was negligible, and she decided to stop taking Celebrex.

For many of my patients, including Maria, supplements have proven to be a critical addition (or supplement, pun intended) to their RA regimen. Like fish oil that helped Maria, supplements aren't like drugs or medications: Before they're released for public use, drugs and medications undergo years of rigorous screening and testing by the FDA. Part of the FDA review of studies includes making sure that the medication is effective for the disease or condition it's supposed to help. On the other hand, supplements, like the kind you buy at the health or grocery store, don't undergo the same regulation process.

As a result, some supplement manufacturing companies use loopholes in federal regulations to market these to the public. This results in the fact that even though a supplement is marketed one way (eg. 'for RA pain') this claim isn't necessarily backed by science.

The loopholes can also impact the quality of a supplement. For example, the FDA has few regulations on who, why, and which ingredients can be labeled natural, meaning that marketing agencies are free to use the term as they please. Many supplements marketed as natural only contain one or two 'natural' ingredients and can contain harmful chemical fillers. So, even if something is labeled 'natural,' it might not be, so keep this in mind as you read and shop.

So there are two things to keep in mind when considering using supplements as part of your RA treatment regimen: 1) Are there well-executed scientific studies that back the effectiveness of the supplement; 2) Is the supplement manufacturer known to use high-quality, non-harmful ingredients?

> ○ PROTIP
> Warning! Supplements are not a substitute for your RA treatment!

During their medical training, doctors aren't taught about the use of supplements. Many physicians never discuss them with their patients or disregard them entirely, telling patients that these won't help their symptoms. This isn't the case, and I'm not "many physicians."

I get it! Many patients, like Maria, are in search of a less toxic, less aggressive intervention for their disease. As a result, many patients take supplements and don't tell their doctor out of fear of ridicule. They will not even tell us due to fear of being ridiculed. They know many traditionally trained physicians advise against taking supplements. As doctors, we must accept a patient's choice and, if the supplement a patient has chosen to use isn't scientifically proven to be effective (or worse yet, if the supplement can cause other problems), advise them against it. This means physicans must conduct more research and guide our patients based on the current scientific evidence. Otherwise, we risk letting our patients get scammed by baseless claims–or hurt by supplements that aren't appropriate for the patient's condition.

> **Not all supplements are natural and not all are safe!**
>
> Supplements, even those marketed as a 'natural alternative,' can be ineffective or even dangerous in high doses. Because they're often sold at grocery stores and pharmacies and don't require a prescription, the general public assumes that all supplements are safe to take. This is not always the case! Before you start any supplement, discuss it with your doctor, as it may result in dangerous drug-to-drug interactions.

The supplements I present in this chapter are recommended to be effective based on thousands of hours of personal research and years of practice. While some can support other conditions as well as RA, fish oil, turmeric, vitamin

D, and probiotics are scientifically proven to help reduce inflammation and the number of swollen and painful joints and improve disease activity. A supplement's dose and, as mentioned, quality, play an essential role in its effects; we'll discuss this in great detail throughout the chapter. And, as always, I'll include action steps to help you determine exactly how much you should take and why.

Fish Oil & Omega-3s

Fish oil and omega-3 supplements are the most popular on the market. The public spends over $2 million on these every year.

Fish oil is extracted from fatty or oily fish, such as **trout, mackerel, tuna, herring, sardines, and salmon**. It is high in omega-3 fatty acids, which yield a variety of health benefits but are especially important for those struggling with RA. Omega-3 fatty acids influence an enzyme called COX-2, the same one blocked by over-the-counter anti inflammatory medications (NSAIDs, such as ibuprofen, naproxen, diclofenac, and meloxicam) that lessen bodily inflammation.

Omega-3s have many health benefits like:
▪ Lower triglyceride levels
▪ Lower blood pressure
▪ Reduced heart rate and heart rate variability
▪ Reduced inflammation.

Fish oil supplements have been shown to significantly improve the symptoms reported by RA patients by decreasing the blood levels of inflammation markers (including TNF-alpha, Interleukin-1, and Interleukin-6 cytokines), all proteins known to produce inflammation in your body.[1] In 2017, a systematic review looked at the benefits of fish oil for arthritis, specifically RA, lupus, gout, and osteoarthritis.[2] Of 22 trials involving RA, almost all found that fish oil—in daily doses ranging from 0.2 to nearly 5 grams of EPA (eicosapentaenoic acid) and 0.2 to 2.1 grams of DHA (docosahexaenoic acid)—significantly reduced joint pain, stiffness, and swelling and reduced or eliminated patients' use of NSAIDs (over-ther-counter ibuprofren or presribed medications such as Ibuprofen, Naproxen or Celebrex).

> ○ **PROTIP**
>
> The recommended daily dose of Fish oil is 2-4 grams. A typical 1,000 mg fish oil supplement contains around 120 mg of DHA and 180 mg of EPA.

Other studies illustrate how slightly more fish oil than recommended by the FDA (5.5 grams as opposed to the 2.5-4 grams recommended by the FDA) can lead to quicker remission and lowered RA disease activity.[3] Better yet, many of these studies reported no additional side effects.

The benefits of omega-3s in RA patients
- Lower duration of morning stiffness
- Fewer tender and swollen joints
- Lower reported levels of overall pain
- Lower fatigue
- Reduced back pain
- Lower use of NSAID medications

Beyond its anti-inflammatory benefits, omega-3s have also been shown to reduce pain. A study of 250 patients with back or neck pain found that, in just four months, 60% of patients discontinued taking their prescription NSAID medications for pain because they didn't need it.[4] NSAIDs (even over-the-counter NSAIDS) are associated with potentially dangerous side effects, like heartburn, stomach ulcers, liver and kidney issues, and even a higher risk of heart attacks. This study is crucial; it suggests omega-3s are comparable to NSAID use without the added harmful side effects.

The omega-3s effect is comparable to NSAID-use without the added harmful side effects.

My recommendation comes with a slight warning: Some fish oil products can be contaminated with mercury. When choosing a supplement, choose one with a sustainability certification, like the Marine Stewardship Council (MSC).

Furthermore, fish oil can potentially decrease your body's absorption of certain medications, so discussing their use with your doctor is essential. Fish oil and omega-3s can interact negatively with blood thinners, blood pressure, or contraceptive medications. If you take them, your doctor should do a blood test to determine your current omega-3 fatty acid levels.

The benefits of omega-3s aren't to be overlooked, especially for RA patients. I recommend taking omega-3 supplements with meals, as other dietary fats improve their absorption (taking fish oil with meals can also prevent stomach upset). Then, start supplementation gradually, with just 1 gram a day for two weeks. If you don't notice any side effects, you can increase your dosage to 2 grams daily to eliminate residual pain and swelling.

Turmeric

In the last chapter, we briefly discussed turmeric, its active ingredient, curcumin, and its role in mitigating persistent RA symptoms. Over 120 clinical studies point to curcumin's impact on our immune system and its antioxidant qualities. In the body, curcumin modulates immune system cells, stopping them from triggering the inflammation and pain caused by RA.[5] Like fish oil and omega-3s, curcumin acts on the COX-2 enzyme, blocking it and fighting pain.

In 2017, a randomized control study on RA patients showed that those who take curcumin experienced a dramatic improvement in their symptoms, including lower inflammation marker levels.[6] Even better—the study found no side effects.

Furthermore, in 2021, a meta-analysis (a review of multiple clinical studies) of RA patients who took curcumin daily for twelve weeks showed the following benefits:[7]

- Decreased joint pain and swelling
- Reduced markers of inflammation and,
- Lower levels of rheumatoid factor

Lessening swelling and joint pain isn't all curcumin can do: Similar to omega-3 fatty acids, research shows that curcumin fights pain just as well as NSAID medications.[8]

> ○ **PROTIP**
>
> Take 1-1.5 grams of turmeric a day for optimal effects. Choose a product enhanced with pepper, which boosts gut absorption. Turmeric contains about 3-8% curcumin (depending on the growing season); 3 g turmeric powder contains an average of 30-90 mg of curcumin.

High doses of curcumin may act as a blood thinner and can potentially increase the activity of any blood-thinning medication (like coumadin or warfarin), increasing your risk for bleeding. As you'll hear me say many times, speaking to a doctor before trying or using curcumin supplements is crucial.

Probiotics

As discussed in the last chapter, probiotics are healthy bacteria intentionally introduced to the gut microbiome to diversify and boost the number of healthy microbes living there.

In recent years, probiotic supplements have become popular due to their notable role in lowering inflammation and inflammation marker levels (such as TNF-alpha, IL-6, and IL-12).

For RA patients specifically, probiotics are a crucial focus: A 2014 study looking at RA patients showed that the introduction of a probiotic (Lactobacillus casei) daily for eight weeks helped significantly decrease joint pain and swelling, decrease stiffness, and lowered the patient's levels of inflammatory markers.[9]

> ○ **PROTIP**
>
> Look for probiotic supplements with 10-20 billion CFU (colonies forming units) and use them for at least eight weeks, then assess the benefits.

In short, probiotics fight inflammation by introducing new, healthy bacteria to the gut, supporting microbial diversity. Because many RA patients suffer from dysbiosis (see chapter 4), probiotics emerge as a potential intervention to help you fight pain, inflammation, and stiffness.

Vitamin D

For years, scientists believed Vitamin D's benefits stopped at calcium absorption, bone growth, and maintenance. We couldn't have been more wrong; vitamin D plays several important functions, including:

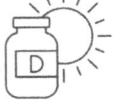

- Antioxidant
- Neuroprotective (fights against injury and damage to your brain and nervous system)
- Muscle maintenance and function
- Anti-inflammatory
- Regulates gut mucosal permeability (the gut lining and what passes through it)

Vitamin D's role as an anti inflammatory render it a powerful supplement for RA patients. Vitamin D affects receptors in your immune and joint cells.[10] Called "vitamin D receptors," these are found in nearly all of your body's immune system cells. Vitamin D interacts with these receptors, regulating the function of T-cells (which can cause or aggravate inflammation) and lowering the number of pro-inflammatory cells in the body. Some studies show active vitamin D (D-3) mediates and regulates our immune system response.

In humans, vitamin D deficiency is associated with
- Type 1 diabetes
- Multiple sclerosis
- Lupus
- Rheumatoid arthritis
- Inflammatory bowel disease
- Depression.

Let's take a look at another fascinating study published in 2022. This study, called the VITAL study, used a randomized, double-blind, controlled trial of 25,000 people to examine the effect of vitamin D and omega-3 fatty acid supplementation.[11,12] After following up a few years later, patients who consumed vitamin D supplements showed a 22% reduction in their risk of developing autoimmune diseases, and those who took a fish oil supplement enjoyed a 15% lowered risk—pretty cool, right?

> ○ **PROTIP**
>
> Experts recommend 2,000 IU of vitamin D daily to reduce the risk of autoimmune disease in people over 50.

Other studies support this: One following the lives of nearly 30,000 women found that those who consumed more vitamin D had a lower risk of developing RA.[13] Others examining patients with the diagnosis showed that the more vitamin D patients consumed, the lower their disease activity.[14]

What is a randomized controlled trial?

A randomized controlled trial is a scientific study where researchers randomly assign participants to different groups. One group receives the tested treatment, while another group (the control group) receives either a standard treatment or a placebo (a dummy treatment with no real effect). The goal is to see if the new treatment works better than the standard treatment or placebo. By randomly assigning participants, researchers can be more confident that any outcome differences are due to the treatment and not other factors. This is the best type of study design for testing a therapy.

How can you get more vitamin D?

Your body's primary source of vitamin D is actually through your skin! In response to UVB exposure, the lower layers of the epidermis produce vitamin D naturally. However, many people avoid the sun due to the increased risk of skin cancer or apply sunscreen that blocks UV light, so it's important to look at food and supplements to get enough to make a difference in your RA.

Because of its role in mediating our immune system response, vitamin D may be a powerful supplement to decrease the risk of developing an autoimmune disease and fight inflammation in those struggling with RA. Research overwhelmingly supports its use, and I regularly test patients' vitamin D blood levels and recommend vitamin D supplementation when appropriate.

> **How to increase your Vitamin D level?**
>
> ACTION STEPS:
>
> 1. Ask your doctor for a baseline vitamin D test. If you learn you're deficient, start supplementation. Then ask for regular monitoring of your vitamin D every six-twelve months.
> 2. Spend at least ten minutes per day in the sun (before applying sunscreen).
> 3. Eat fish at least three times per week.
> 4. Add vitamin D-fortified products to your diet (milk, cheese, cereals).

Other Supplements That Fight RA Symptoms

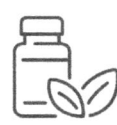

Though I recommend that those struggling with painful RA symptoms give fish oil, turmeric, probiotics, and vitamin D a try, these aren't the only supplements I found scientific evidence for that might be of help. I scoured Pubmed, the world's most extensive online medical library, for other supplements that alleviate RA symptoms.

I discuss some of these supplements and studies in depth in my online course; here, I'll provide a brief overview.

Quercetin is a flavonoid known for its antiinflammatory and antioxidant benefits. Studies in RA patients who used a Quercetin supplement (500 mg/day for 8 weeks) found significantly less pain and stiffness and lower levels of inflammatory markers.[15,16] Additionally, quercetin can lessen bone loss. This is crucial for RA patients whose above-average risk of bone weakening leaves them susceptible to osteoporosis and damage.

Pomegranate extract is another compelling option for those struggling with joint pain from RA. Pomegranate seeds contain antioxidants and polyphenols, which can help prevent free radicals from damaging cells. Free radicals are unstable molecules produced in the body in response to many things, from exposure to toxins like cigarette smoke, as well as stress. One randomized control study published in *Nature*, a highly respected medical journal, reported that patients with RA who received a pomegranate extract supplement (500 mg daily) for 12 weeks enjoyed drastic symptom improvement, including less joint pain and fewer bodily free radicals.[17]

Garlic has been used medicinally since ancient times. Proven to benefit those with heart disease and diabetes, studies similarly corroborate garlic's benefits for RA patients. One study on RA patients found that consumption of an aged garlic supplement (3.6 grams per day for 6 weeks) decreased a patient's number of swollen and painful joints, fatigue, and improved disease activity measures.[18]

Sesamin is a compound naturally found in sesame oil. Sesamin yields an anti-inflammatory effect by influencing the COX-2 enzyme, which we've discussed in other sections, and by lessening inflammatory marker levels. Furthermore, sesamin reduces levels of specific enzymes (such as hyaluronidase and matrix metalloproteinases-3) involved in joint destruction, a common problem in RA. A 2019 study of RA patients found that those taking a sesamin supplement (200 mg daily for six weeks) enjoyed significantly improved swelling and joint pain compared to those who didn't.[19]

CoQ10 enzyme is an antioxidant naturally found in your body's cells. It's a substance that converts the food you eat into energy and bears powerful effects on your circulatory and immune systems. For example, CoQ10 can potentially lower your risk of developing heart disease, high blood pressure, and periodontal disease, all of which often occur concurrently with RA. Zooming in on RA specifically, this enzyme (100 mg taken daily) has been shown to reduce bodily inflammation.[20] Additionally, the CoQ10 enzyme can lower your pain score and the number of swollen and tender joints you're experiencing.

Ginger has been used for centuries both as a spice and for its medicinal properties. As we discussed in Chapter 5, ginger is a pain-reliever: One study found that 1500 mg of ginger supplementation (taken over 12 weeks) reduced RA patients' pain and lessened their reliance on rescue medications or over-the-counter painkillers.[21]

Boswellia is the resin from the Boswellia tree. Boswellic acids, one of the compounds found in Boswellia, have anti-inflammatory properties.[22] Like fish oil/omega-3s and curcumin, boswellic acids block the same enzymes as NSAIDs, decreasing inflammation and reducing cartilage damage. While there are many studies illustrating the benefits of Boswellia supplements in people with osteoarthritis, evidence remains sparse for RA patients specifically. Most studies reporting benefits were done in animals and not humans. Boswellia use comes with a warning: These supplements can negatively interact with other drugs, such as antidepressants, anti-anxiety medications, ibuprofen, and immunosuppressants, which can increase your risk of side effects.

Collagen peptides (or collagen hydrolysate) are one of the most common supplements advertised for people with arthritis. Many studies have reported positive results for patients with osteoarthritis, including less pain, stiffness, and improved physical function. However, in patients with RA, the effect of collagen peptides is still debatable. Collagen might have some anti-inflammatory properties that are helpful for patients with RA, but there's insufficient evidence of benefit. While collagen supplements might not be harmful, especially for those struggling with osteoarthritis, there isn't enough evidence to determine whether it can help RA patients specifically.

Get Started with Supplements

The supplements I've introduced in this chapter are a powerful intervention for RA patients, particularly those who continue to struggle with painful and swollen joints, fatigue, and morning stiffness. Some, like fish oil, turmeric, and sesamin, influence the same enzyme as pain-reliever medications, positively influencing a patient's pain and disease activity levels. Others, like vitamin D, moderate the body's inflammatory response, lessening pain. Nevertheless, these supplements are scientifically proven to help you find relief.

How do you make sure you get a quality supplement?

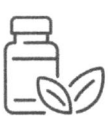

The best way to ensure the quality of a supplement product is to look for one with a third-party certification that will provide the supplement-producing company with a Certificate of Analysis (COA). This COA will ensure the consumer that ingredients listed on the bottle are included, that ingredients and doses remain the same between different batches, and that there are no contaminants like heavy metals or other toxins in the product. Some of these certifications include NSF, USP, and ConsumerLab. Look out for these when purchasing a new supplement.

I recommend each of these supplements conditionally: Along with your conventional medication, each has been proven to provide RA patients solace from pesky pain and inflammation. Keep in mind that these won't and can't replace your prescribed RA treatment, as much as you may want them to. If you're ready to try these, discuss them with your doctor and take the appropriate doses. Check out the side boxes for information on how to get started, and find relief!

How to start supplementation? Step-by-step guide:

1. Discuss your interest in supplements with your doctor, and ask them to check for potential drug interactions.
2. Before starting a supplement, assess your pain levels, number of swollen and painful joints and inflammation markers levels. (*In my practice, I usually check a patient's blood work before they begin a supplement, and re-check at regular intervals)
3. As with any supplement, start slow. Increase your dosage gradually while monitoring for side effects.
4. If you experience side effects, stop taking the supplement immediately.
5. Don't start multiple supplements at the same time. That way, you can pinpoint which one is causing your side effects.
6. Re-evaluate the supplement's effect every two to three months. You may continue if you notice improvements in joint pain or fewer swollen joints. If there is no improvement, consider stopping the supplement.

CHAPTER 7

IT'S NOT IN YOUR HEAD: STRESS, RA, AND HEALING

When I met thirty-eight-year-old Sophia in my office three years ago, she greeted me with hope and frustration. "Dr. G," she told me. "You're the third rheumatologist I've seen. The other doctors say that what I have is fibromyalgia, but I want another perspective on my case."

She told me that she'd been in pain for about 18 months. Besides that, she was healthy and had never taken any medication before. I examined her and ordered regular tests but found that her rheumatoid factor and anti-CCP antibody tests were both negative, which confused me a little. I understood why other physicians thought she had fibromyalgia, but something about that didn't seem right; I ordered an MRI of her hands, saw some damage to her joints, and concluded that Sophia suffered from seronegative Rheumatoid arthritis, a form of arthritis where the regular tests (rheumatoid factor and anti-CCP antibodies) were negative (Remember our discussion in Chapter 3; about 20% of patients with RA have negative blood tests). We initiated treatment, and within months, Sophia felt significantly better and reported less pain and swelling in her hands.

However, during one visit, she paused and asked me "I know I've gotten much better—the pain is much more manageable, and I feel less stiff in the morning. But I'm not sure—something still isn't quite right."

I asked, "What makes you say that?"

She hesitated and took some time to explain herself. "I don't know. I feel like I'm doing better, but on certain days I feel like I've taken three steps backward. My pain is worse than it was even before treatment, and I can't seem to get out of bed in the morning."

Knowing what I do about the connection between the body and the brain, I decided to probe further. "What's different about those days, Sophia?" I asked her.

"I'm not sure—they're just days," she told me, shrugging her shoulders.

"Is anything different on those days you feel more pain? What about the day before?" Sophia shrugged again, not wanting to answer the question.

I decided to talk with her about the connection between the body and brain: "The mind and body are intimately connected, and often, stress in one causes pain in the other," I explained, motioning with my hands.

"Come on, Dr. G," she chuckled. "You don't expect me to believe this is all in my head, do you?"

"This isn't all in your head," I told her, taking her hands. "What's happening in the brain can cause physical changes to the body. Stress can worsen pain—it's science," I said.

Sophia rolled her eyes. "You're just trying to make me feel better."

"Well yes," I am, I told her, chuckling. "That's my job. But you know I would never mention anything that isn't backed by science."

She shook her head. "I mean—I'm stressed. But isn't everyone?" she asked.

"Not necessarily," I told her. "What's going on at home?"

Sophia began to tell me more about her life: Her last five years were stressful. She was the primary caregiver to a child who suffered a severe, rare genetic disease, and she'd lost her sister, with whom she was close. Tears welled in her eyes as she finished, saying, "And after all that, my marriage is suffering. My partner says that I'm just not here anymore."

I grabbed her hands in mine. "Sophia, your observations aren't just in your head. This stress is likely causing your RA to worsen." She shrugged again, still apprehensive.

The Mind-Body Connection

We tend to think of the two—the mind and the body—as separate entities. Many doctors are no exception to this "we."

But this is a fallacy: More and more research shows that the mind and the body are deeply reliant on one another. A pain, ache, or stiffness in the body impacts the mind, and thoughts, feelings, and emotions in the mind affect your pain. These thoughts, feelings, and emotions aren't transient reactions but embodied by your gut, limbs, and chest. Feelings live within us, and it's essential to attend to them.

The brain is responsible for this connection: Contrary to what scientists believed years ago, the brain isn't simply your body's engine but your body's life force. It's a remarkably complex organ, harboring your thoughts, feelings, and emotions and commanding your bodily functions, including walking, talking, and digestion.

Furthermore, many of these functions are mediated by neurochemicals and hormones. Take emotions, for example: The neurochemicals and hormones released and absorbed by the brain control what we feel, be it happy, sad, or angry. These neurochemicals and hormones also affect our blood pressure, heart rate, sleep, and appetite—hence why you may feel hungry in response to a loss, rejection, or boredom.

Recently, researchers at Washington University in St. Louis took a closer look at the mind-body connection, building brain maps using MRI technology.[1] The study used color to illustrate the brain's connections—the more intense the color, the stronger the connections are. In bright, vibrant shades, they found that areas of the brain previously thought to control only heart rate and essential bodily functions also lit up in response to thinking and planning, illustrating connectedness. Lead researcher Dosenbach said of the results, "All of these connections make sense if you think about what the brain is really for," Dosenbach said. "You move your body for a reason… Pain is the most powerful feedback. You do something, and it hurts, and you think, 'I'm not doing that again.'"

In the gut microbiome chapter, we discussed the gut-mind connection, and the gut's role in regulating our bodily functions, such as appetite, digestion, mood, and, very importantly for RA patients, immune system functioning. We discussed how anxiety causes butterflies in your stomach, but this is just one tactile example of your mind and body's interconnectedness. Feelings of heartache in response to grief or loss, shaky hands before a big test or interview, or a headache after you receive lousy news are each examples of how your mind and body communicate—or talk—to one another throughout the day. Studies point to emotions most prominently affecting these three key processes: The immune response, digestion, and wound healing.

Joint damage, a form of wound, is the 'tip of the iceberg' for RA patients. For those struggling with RA, understanding the mind-body connection and stress's role in their health is paramount to breaking the vicious cycle in their gut, body, and mind. In this chapter, we'll discuss how to manage stress and promote relaxation to help the mind and the body, leaving them with less inflammation and pain.

A Vicious Cycle: Stress & the Immune System

All of us are a little stressed out. But stress, in its natural form, isn't necessarily bad. Some forms of stress, or *good stress*, can be helpful and motivating. Let's say you have a significant, looming deadline at work tomorrow, and you sit down and work on your proposal for a few hours in response. This type of stress, called *eustress*, is relatively positive—it motivates you to get things done.

Unfortunately, *bad stress* is much more common: Bad stress is the thoughts running through your brain on your drive home from work—you're thinking, "I can't possibly meet this deadline," "The kids needed to be picked up five minutes ago," or, "Oh crap—I forgot to defrost the chicken for dinner." These are small examples, but this kind of stress—*bad stress*— isn't positive at all and yields no motivation or results. In fact, many of us find it debilitating.

Bad stress isn't just harmful emotionally, but rather physically. The American Academy of Family Physicians recently reported that, in the past twenty years, 66% of medical visits are the cause of stress-related symptoms, such as heart issues, stomach discomfort, and chronic pain. Additionally, 33% of patients who go to the ER with chest pain are found to have minimal heart issues–their arteries are blockage-free and are instead found to have panic attacks, which is causing their discomfort.

But why is this the case? Stress activates your body's sympathetic nervous system, known as your "fight or flight" response. This response releases stress hormones, including cortisol and adrenaline, responsible for the physical feeling of panic—increased heart rate, high blood pressure, sweating—that you experience in response to a stressful thought or event.

The cardiovascular system isn't the only one responding to these hormones: Your immune system reacts, increasing inflammation to maximize immunity to what your body perceives as a danger. In small doses, these stress hormones are protective and improve immune function. Still, in large doses, as is the case in chronic stress, the constant release of cortisol and adrenaline disrupts nearly all of your bodily systems—over 75% of chronic diseases are related to the body's stress response.[2]

Cortisol is so powerful that it can lower a person's white blood cell response (a component of our immune response) to cancer cells and viruses.[3] In stressed people, vaccinations are less effective, and wounds don't heal as well as they usually would.

> O **PROTIP**
>
> Chronic stress lowers your immune system and response to vaccines, and decreases your wound healing.

Prolonged high cortisol levels cause an uptick in inflammatory markers and cytokines such as IL-6, TNF-a, and CRP, which suppress the immune system. Over time, this increases your likelihood of developing infections and autoimmune diseases like RA.[2]

This isn't the only problem with stress. Stress is anxiety's precursor: Anxiety refers to your body and mind's reaction to a specific stressor—to whatever is stressing you out. Looking at RA specifically, if you're stressed about the morning stiffness you feel when you get out of bed, anxiety is the racing thoughts that follow, like:

"Why is this happening to me?" or,

"Will this disease take over my body?"

"Will I get disabled and lose my independence?"

When I welcome a new patient into my practice, I often allow them time to share their story—whatever that means to them. Many patients tell me about a recent divorce, losing someone they loved, changing jobs, moving into a new home, or surgery—each stressful life event. Like Sophia, soon after these stressful events, the pain, swelling, and stiffness in their joints become more evident. Even if they had similar episodes of pain in the past, these become more frequent, more acute, and more debilitating, causing them to come to my office asking for help.

Does Stress Cause RA?

As a physician, I'm happy to explain the importance of the mind, body, and connection to my patients, especially skeptics like Sophia. Because of this connection, stress in our minds affects vital bodily systems. So, for RA patients, it seems prudent to discuss stress's role. Unfortunately, this conversation is all too rare in rheumatology offices, but with this knowledge, you can unlock your mind and learn to use it as a tool to mitigate your RA symptoms.

But more and more research is also revealing that stress–especially chronic, long-term stress, may also be a contributing factor to whether a person develops RA or not. Interestingly, recent research shows that stress is linked to developing RA. For example, women who have PTSD, or post-traumatic stress disorder, are at two times the risk of developing RA.[4] Even women who've suffered from the perceived stress of inflammatory arthritis (meaning they're afraid of having the disease but haven't received a formal diagnosis) develop increased levels of inflammation and become at risk of developing RA, the disease they were so afraid of in the first place.[5]

Throughout my years of practice, I've seen many patients stress themselves out over diseases they aren't sure they have! Stress can cause inflammation, so I recommend that all patients take a little breather regardless of their diagnosis status. Stressing yourself out won't help! Leave it to your specialist or rheumatologist—they can sort out your diagnosis.

Stress & RA: The Last Piece of the Puzzle

Now that we understand and recognize that stress is a critical factor that can increase your risk of developing RA, let's talk about how stress affects people suffering from the illness itself.

As you already know, living with RA poses daily challenges: Patients deal with constant joint pain, fatigue, and disability. Some lose their independence as they're unable to be as active as they were before, worry about medical costs and miss time at work. Many patients report trying—and failing—to juggle frequent visits to the doctor and complex treatment programs. Even worse, this can cause issues in a marriage or relationship, as a partner might not understand what you're truly going through.

You can clearly see what I'm getting at here—all of these can cause more STRESS!

Research shows that RA patients have higher cortisol levels when compared to a baseline.[6] In other words, they experience stress at higher levels compared to those who don't suffer from the disease. This stress response causes an increased white blood cell count (immune system cells) and increased inflammation (high levels of TNF-alpha, C-reactive protein), leading to more substantial active disease and pain.[7] In other words, the more stress you experience, the more pain you'll feel, creating a vicious cycle that needs to be stopped.

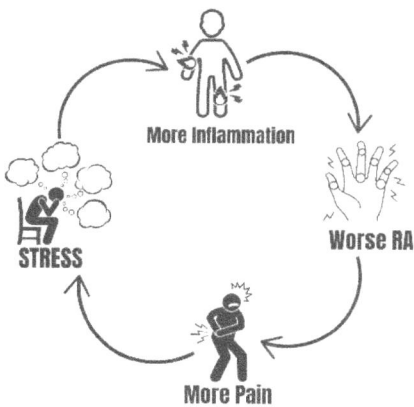

Figure 3. The effect of stress on inflammation and Rheumatoid arthritis

Fight the Stress

The relationship between stress and RA is cyclical: Chronic stress causes inflammation, leading to worsened symptoms and disease activity. On the flip side, RA itself is a stressful condition; navigating complicated treatment protocols and appointments is inherently stressful. Furthermore, few doctors understand stress's role and impact on symptoms, resulting in sparse information about managing it. Worse, all of this aggravates pain, inflammation, and (you guessed it)---stress!

Eliminating stress from our lives is nearly impossible—it's a natural response to keep us safe. Because of this, I tell my patients that *how* we react to stress is more important than *eliminating* it. Learning how to manage stress in RA is essential, and doing so will decrease inflammation, lower your pain, minimize the frequency of your RA flare-ups, and improve your sleep quality (we will address this aspect more in Chapter 9).

You can't eliminate the stress in your life, but you can learn how to react to the stressors in your life.

Recognizing your stressors and triggers, taking steps to mitigate them, and using effective coping strategies such as mindfulness, meditation, breathing techniques, and gratitude journaling (all of which we'll discuss in sections to come) can help you effectively manage your stress and, by proxy, your RA.

Mindfulness: A Key Stress-busting Intervention

In the last section, we explored stress and anxiety's role in your RA and overall health. However, we have a few unanswered questions: "What can I do to fix it?" and, "How on *earth* do I lower my stress?" In this section, as well as those to come, I'll introduce some proven skills, tips, and changes you can make to offset your stress levels and live pain-free.

One of these I highly recommend is mindfulness. Mindfulness is a form of meditation practice rooted in Buddhist and Hindu teachings. Initially, mindfulness intended to cultivate a sense of awareness and wisdom of the world around us, but today, it helps people and patients live through the moments of their lives to the fullest extent possible.

> It's important to note that many people use mindfulness and meditation interchangeably. In this book, however, we'll separate the two.

You've heard of active listening before, the practice of asking questions while remaining open and cultivating positive body language while another is speaking. Similarly, *mindfulness is an attention to the present*. Instead of using another person as your primary focal point, your focal point is your thoughts, actions, and the world around you. Those practicing mindfulness pay active attention to the world around them and observe their thoughts as they arise without judging them positively or negatively. This is important! *The goal is to simply observe your thoughts—do not judge them!*

Those practicing mindfulness don't ignore their distracting thoughts, sensations, and physical discomforts but instead focus on them intently. They look, accept, and learn to welcome their tensions, stress, and pain. Mindfulness practitioners accept the present moment as neither good nor bad, which is a crucial step to healing mentally and physically.

Mindfulness & Medicine: Does It Actually Work?

to Sophia's story, which we began in the previous section (the Mind and Body Connection). Stress caused Sophia's pain to worsen and seemed to trigger her flare-ups. I asked her, "Have you ever heard about mindfulness?"

Sophia nodded and said, "Yeah, but I thought that was like some woo-woo yoga thing. That can't help, can it?"

I nodded and laughed at the comparison. Over the next 30 minutes, I gave Sophia a crash course into mindfulness and provided her with some resources to start incorporating it into her routine. She was skeptical, unsure whether this would work, but for the next few weeks, she began her day with ten minutes of mindful meditation.

At our next appointment, I introduced her to more mindfulness techniques like square breathing and others (all of which we'll discuss throughout this section and chapter). I also asked Sophia to start writing in a daily gratitude journal.

In six months, she came back to my office for a follow-up appointment, and told me that her pain was so much better! "That stuff *actually* worked," she told me with a half-smile. "I can focus at work now, help my child, and my relationship with my husband is much better."

I tell you Sophia's story with a smile and a warm heart; she is just one of many success stories I could provide. Based on how mindfulness has transformed the lives of my patients, I truly believe that mindfulness is an effective tool for patients struggling with any kind of chronic pain, but particularly pain from RA.

Better yet, mindfulness's efficacy is scientifically backed: More than 40 years ago, Dr. Jon Kabat Zin at the University of Massachusetts conducted a study on the effects of mindfulness on patients with chronic pain and inflammation. After just eight weeks of practicing mindfulness, the patients in his research showed dramatic improvements in their pain levels, fatigue, and overall quality of life. For the first time in medical history, Dr. Zin's research proved that mindfulness was an effective way to counteract symptoms. In 1979, Dr. Zin started a stress clinic known as the MBSR (*Mindfulness-Based Stress Reduction*) program, and its teachings have spread globally, incorporated by world-renowned institutions like Stanford University, Harvard University, and Mayo Clinic.

Beyond Dr. Zin's research, many studies illustrate mindfulness's profound effects on the brain and body. In fact, just eight weeks of mindfulness changes the brain structurally by boosting activity in the areas of the brain responsible for self-regulation, attention, test performance, and decision-making.[8] Mindfulness was also shown to influence areas of the brain *linked to perception and pain tolerance and reducing chronic stress.*

Practicing mindfulness grows the hippocampus, the seahorse-shaped area just inside each temple (on both sides of the brain) associated with memory and emotions. Likewise, stress shrinks the hippocampus: Those with chronic stress, PTSD, or depression tend to have a smaller hippocampus. Practicing mindfulness can decrease stress levels, causing the hippocampus to grow back to its normal size.

In response to mindfulness, the amygdala also shrinks (as the hippocampus grows). This is a good thing, as the amygdala is the part of the brain responsible for your fear or anxiety, causing fewer feelings of fear.

Mindfulness's benefits impact the entire body. The practice is linked to an overall better quality of life, reduced mortality in those with heart disease, and decreased pain in patients with inflammatory arthritis, osteoarthritis, fibromyalgia, psoriasis, or inflammatory bowel disease (IBS).

Mindfulness's effect on the body
- Reduces heart rate and blood pressure
- Improves digestion
- Lowers reactivity, anxiety, stress, fear, and anger
- Improves sleep quality
- Enhances immune system
- Decreases inflammation

Looking at RA specifically, scientific studies show that mindfulness drastically benefits patients. A meta-analysis published in 2018 showed that patients with RA practicing mindfulness enjoyed a reduction in overall disease activity. Furthermore, the study found that mindfulness improved patient's depression and stress levels.[9] This isn't the only study showcasing compelling benefits: Another study found that RA patients practicing mindfulness have less pain and a better quality of life.[10]

The benefits of mindfulness in RA patients
- Decreased disease activity
- Improved depression
- Improved anxiety levels
- Decreased pain
- Reduced perception of pain
- Increased tolerance to pain
- Better quality of life

Mindfulness doesn't only benefit your swelling and inflammation: Some of the most substantial evidence proving mindfulness's effectiveness illustrates its role in mitigating pain. Chronic or prolonged pain negatively affects the body and your thoughts. It causes anxiety and depression and is linked to excessive use of opioid medications. Mindfulness has also been shown to influence areas of the brain *related to perception and pain tolerance* and serves as a potent tool for curbing chronic pain. For example, a 2017 study found that mindfulness, yoga, and stress reduction techniques can lower a patient's pain perception, boost mobility, improve bodily functioning, and enhance their sense of well-being.[11]

Learn how to change your relationship with pain: Instead of running from it, you should accept it.

While mindfulness may not alleviate pain entirely, it will help you understand and develop an awareness and tolerance for your pain. Let's say you have pain in your knuckles—this is a common spot of discomfort for RA patients. Paying attention to this painful sensation in your hands allows you to investigate it consciously, explore it, and see it for what it is, not what you think it might become. Noting your sensations, such as a warming or hot feeling, allows you to accept them. In short, understanding and acknowledging pain takes away its power and, thus, your fear.

We must learn to change our relationship with pain: Instead of running from it, we should accept it. When we ruminate about our pain, we ascribe new emotions—frustration, bitterness, sadness, and anger—to it, complicating it, and in turn, making it worse.

> **The parable of the second arrow**
>
> One day a man went to see Buddha. At the time, he was very depressed and many significant, stressful things were happening in his life.
>
> Buddha asked him what was happening, and the man replied, "I have so many problems. Situations only seem to get worse! What's happening to me–why?"
>
> Then, Buddha replied, "Picture yourself walking through a forest. Suddenly, you're hit by an arrow, and it hurts. But, your pain isn't over—soon, you're hurt by a second arrow. How do you think that will feel?"
>
> "It's going to hurt more," said the man.
>
> "In life, we can't always control the first arrow. That is the pain. However the second arrow is our reaction to the first one, and our reaction is optional—we choose how to react."
>
> <u>Teaching Point:</u> The first arrow is inevitable: It is the bad event happening in our life, whether it be divorce, a sick child, the loss of a job or loved one, or chronic pain from RA. This arrow is the physical pain that our bodies respond to. However, the second arrow is suffering—it's emotional pain.
>
> Luckily, we choose how we respond to emotional pain. As Buddha said, an "uninstructed man" will react in two ways: by obsessing, worrying, and wondering what's wrong with him and by blaming himself or others and feeling angry, frustrated, or irritated. The second way the "uninstructed man" responds is through avoidance: He will ignore, avoid, and suppress. However, both of these ways only yield more suffering and pain.
>
> So—what can you do? The third option, or the one used by what Buddha calls the 'instructed man,' is called "Turning Towards." In mindfulness teachings, "Turning Towards" means embracing, allowing, and opening yourself up to an event in your life. We approach it rather than avoid it. Ultimately, it's better to accept pain as a part of your disease and to develop self-compassion than to suffer.
>
> As Budda said, *"Pain is inevitable, but suffering is optional."*

A dear friend shared this story with me, and I've begun sharing *The Parable of the Second Arrow* with my patients. Many find it a helpful way to think about their symptoms.

We can't avoid pain from the first arrow, but we *can* control pain from the second one. So, when you're in pain, allow yourself to feel it. You might feel frustration, irritation, and emotional pain. Notice these reactions—these are the second arrow. Catch yourself adding more pain and suffering and avoid the second arrow.

Pain is inevitable, but suffering is optional.

Be mindful of your pain, but don't let it take your power. You are more than your pain—acknowledge that.

Your Mindfulness Journey: The Beginning

As we discussed in this chapter, for RA patients, mindfulness decreases pain levels and perception while increasing pain tolerance. Because of this research, mindfulness is no longer a "nice to have" habit but rather a must-have skill.

Check out the box to learn more about mindfulness, and most importantly, how to get started. Like Sophia, it's okay to be a little skeptical, but mindfulness isn't silly—its anti-inflammatory and pain-relieving benefits are backed by science.

The 5 steps for pain awareness

The Five Steps for Pain Awareness is a five-step model for mindfulness found and adapted from the book *Living Well with Pain and Illness* by Vidyamala Burch. Follow this exercise to gain a stronger sense of your thoughts and pain.

STEP 1: Awareness—your starting point

First, bring yourself into the present moment. Notice where you are—your setting—and what's around you. Consider what your hands touch; notice noises you hear outside or around you. Ask yourself the following questions:

- What are you saying to yourself?
- What do you feel?
- Do you feel upset, sad, frustrated, or enjoy this moment?
- What physical sensations are you experiencing?

- Do you feel muscle tightness? Are there any painful joints?

Take a deep breath, or pay attention to your breath without trying to change it.

STEP 2 - Move toward the unpleasant

Most people react to pain in one of two ways: We try to block it to distract ourselves from the discomfort, or we drown in the discomfort and associated fear (ex., Asking yourself, "When will this pain end?").

Today, you have a third option: Rather than distracting yourself or drowning it out, notice your pain. Move your attention to it and ask yourself the following:

- What am I feeling? Is this a burning, cutting, or aching pain?
- Where do I experience the pain?
- Where does the pain start?
- Where does the pain end?

STEP 3 - Seeking the pleasant

Pain affects us physically and mentally, impacting our thoughts. This critical step invites you to find something pleasant about your present experience. Think of it like an exploration—you're searching around a cavern for hidden treasure. Your pleasantness might be a shallow breath, warm hands, or a pleasant feeling in your stomach.

STEP 4- Broadening awareness

It's time to include both the pleasant and the unpleasant in your experience. Your body is a whole entity, consisting of contrasting feelings all at once and all the time. Consider and rest your mind on your whole body, not just those areas that cause you pain. You are much bigger than one or the other. Include your surroundings in your meditation, noticing pleasant things in your environment, the softness of a pillow or blanket, the sound of birds or a fountain, or a pleasant smell.

STEP 5 -Your choice

Respond to what you're feeling—don't just react to it. Move your attention to the world around you. Allow yourself to respond, not just react to what you're feeling. Aim to control your thoughts and maintain your curiosity.

Now, pause for a moment. You might be surprised by what happens next!

Ommm, Ommm: Reclaim Your Body with Meditation

Think back to the last section: Meditation was one of the interventions I offered Sophia. While she was initially skeptical, she gleaned meditation's vast benefits: Less stress, pain, inflammation, and morning stiffness. This section will discuss the tools and tips I gave Sophia to help you reap the same compelling results.

Like Sophia, many patients seem a little skeptical when I discuss with them the transformative power of meditation on their RA symptoms: They tell me that there is no way focusing on one thing for a few minutes a day could really help them, and to this, I tell them to try it. Check out the table below for a few more common myths I often hear.

Common myths and misconceptions surrounding meditation

Common Myths	Truth
Myth 1. **Meditation is difficult.**	Don't consider meditation an out-of-touch, intangible practice reserved for only monks living on a hill. Meditation is easy and relatively fun. Some meditation techniques are more advanced than others, so don't dive into a meditative feast on your first try! Instead, start by silently repeating a word or mantra, focusing on your breath, and closing your eyes. Focus on the practice itself—not a preconceived idea of the perfect end result.
Myth 2: **You must stop thinking for a successful meditation session.**	Meditation isn't about "emptying" your mind or stopping your thoughts. We can't control our thoughts, but we can decide how much attention we should give them. People teaching meditation techniques often suggest "noticing thoughts," then letting them float by. Through meditation, you'll learn to find the gap between your thoughts—within this gap are pure consciousness, silence, and peace.
Myth 3. **It takes years to see benefits.**	Meditation holds both immediate and long-term benefits. Many people, even after just a few days, begin feeling these benefits gradually. Studies conducted at both Harvard and the University of Massachusetts show that just eight weeks of MBSR programming has profound benefits and effects on the brain's structure, yielding emotional clarity, reducing stress, and improving sleep quality.
Myth 4. **I don't have enough time to meditate.**	You don't need to spend hours on meditation—for most people, it takes just a few minutes (even only 10 minutes a day strongly impacts your stress and pain levels).
Myth 5. **Meditation requires certain spiritual and religious beliefs.**	Meditation doesn't require a specific spiritual belief. Meditation, in various forms, is present in nearly all major world religions, including Christianity and Judaism. Many people can practice and benefit from meditation, regardless of their reason for doing so. Make yourself your reason. You can thank me later!

Meditation, another hallmark of Buddhist practice and principles, refers to a variety of practices that you can use to calm your mind and improve your overall well-being.[12] In fact, meditation yields several positive benefits, including more positive moods, lessened pain, increased concentration, and stronger feelings of social connection. Physically, meditation has been shown to reduce inflammation and pain and can help those suffering from IBS, fibromyalgia, and (you guessed it!) Rheumatoid arthritis.

Like mindfulness, some of the most substantial evidence for meditation lies in its potential for pain relief. One study of chronic pain patients found that, after an eight-week meditation program, patients experienced significant improvements in their anxiety, depressive symptoms, and pain levels.[13] In fact, those who are chronically stressed show a higher response rate to meditation than those who experience lower amounts of stress.

But what about you? A 2022 systematic literature review looked exclusively at the potential impact of meditation, mindfulness, and yoga (see the last section for more details about mindfulness more specifically) on RA patients' health and overall wellbeing.[14]

The conclusion?

Meditation helped RA patients improve their physical functioning and overall health. Both resulted in improved quality of life scores compared to those who didn't try the intervention.

In short, meditation offers those suffering from RA less pain and acts as a mediator for much of the pain you're experiencing. I highly recommend giving it a try to reduce your symptom's severity and alleviate your pain.

How to Practice Meditation?

Meditation is a relatively simple practice and requires minimal time investment. Follow these steps and try them to begin incorporating meditation (and mindfulness) into your day:

While mindfulness and meditation often overlap, they are different practices for your mind.

1. Allot yourself for five to ten minutes, and find a quiet space to engage in your meditation practice. Make sure you're in a space that feels uplifting, whether it be your couch, carpet, or near a window. Do your best to eliminate distractions.

2. Take a moment to find a posture that feels "right" for you. Your position should feel relaxed and dignified. Sit either cross-legged or upright.
3. Keep your eyes open, and rest them downward—either on an object or floor—approximately five feet before you.
4. Find an object of attention, whether it be the thing you're looking at, your breath, a mental image, or a relaxing mantra (this is concentration).
5. Notice and pay attention to your breath. Let the air flow through your nose, into your lungs and chest, and then back out your mouth.
6. As you think, notice your thoughts: Don't judge or push them away. When you feel a thought or sensation pulling you away from the present, return to the present moment. Again—don't judge; note (that this overlaps with the mindfulness practice we discussed before).
7. End the session after the first five to ten minutes; then don't speed back into life just yet—take a few moments to live in the peace you've created for yourself.

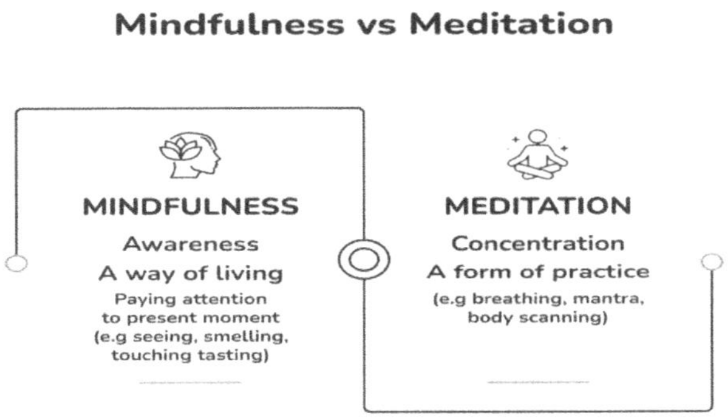

Mindfulness vs Meditation

MINDFULNESS	MEDITATION
Awareness	Concentration
A way of living	A form of practice
Paying attention to present moment (e.g seeing, smelling, touching tasting)	(e.g breathing, mantra, body scanning)

Figure 4. The difference between Mindfulness and Meditation

As I tell my patients, we prioritize what's important to us, so make meditation a priority. As you stick to your routine and build time for meditation into your day, you'll notice your focus improving, and you can accomplish much more in less time.

> **My best advice**
>
> *Hold no expectations for yourself.* Sometimes, your mind will be active throughout your session, and during others, it won't. Remember, *mindfulness is a practice, not a performance.*
>
> *Second, find a technique that works for you.* Your mind is unique! The method I mentioned is just one of thousands, so don't be afraid to consult Google, YouTube, Spotify, or Audible to find guided meditation practices.
>
> *Finally, be there in the moment.* Ensure you're alone when you meditate, and *turn off all devices before you begin.* If other thoughts arise, acknowledge them and move on.

Meditation is a crucial stress-reducing intervention for RA patients. Not only will it reduce your pain and inflammation, but it's scientifically proven to improve your quality of life drastically.

On my YouTube channel, I offer a video with positive, empowering affirmations. Check out the resource section of this book for more information, and get started with meditation today!

Breathing Better

Breathing is a complex process involving the brain, lungs, respiratory muscles, diaphragm, and red blood cells (which carry the oxygen we inhale to our body's cells and organs).

Breathing keeps us alive—we can't live without it!

Our bodies breathe through our mouth and nose, which travels down to our lungs. The lungs deliver oxygen to the rest of the body through our circulatory system. As a result, breathing affects our autonomic nervous system (the part of the nervous system that regulates involuntary processes, such as heart rate, blood pressure and the like, and the vagus nerve). As we briefly noted in earlier chapters, the vagus nerve affects our emotions, blood pressure, heart rate, inflammation, and digestion.[15] It also connects our ears, vocal cords, heart, lungs, and intestines.

> Did you Know that we breathe in and out approximately 22,000 times daily?

Conscious reathing (also known as breathwork) can impact the vagus nerve and lower your heart rate. Here's how it works: Slow, deep nasal breathing engages the diaphragm, which is connected with the vagus nerve and also to your heart. When you exhale, the vagus nerve activates the parasympathetic nervous system, which is responsible for decreasing the heart rate and calming you down.[16] This gives us a moment to chill out, so to speak.

Most of us aren't aware of our breathing, at least not until it becomes difficult for us to do so. This kind of breathing, which you don't have to think about, is called unconscious breathing. While unconscious breathing is what you need to survive, *mindful breathing*, or *conscious breathing*, is what's necessary to keep your RA symptoms at bay. *Mindful breathing* is the kind you think about and is responsible for stress, cortisol levels, anxiety, and pain.

> Unconscious Breathing (the breathing that you do not think about) vs Conscious / Mindful breathing (the action of breathing that you think about).

Recently, scientists examining the power of conscious breath and the vagus nerve discovered that applying short spurts of electrical stimulation to the vagus nerve activates a new neural pathway that decreases inflammation in RA patients.[17] This research is exciting and could be applied to patients with Sjogren's syndrome, lupus, osteoarthritis, and fibromyalgia. Finally, we understand the pivotal role our breathing plays in inflammation and pain.[18]

> If you're interested in learning more about these studies, check out this website for updated information: https://reset-ra.study/

Don't fear—if you don't have access to these treatments, there are other, more accessible ways to stimulate the vagus nerve. In truth, *mindful breathing* is simple—focus solely on your breath. As you do so, consider its natural flow, thinking about each inhale and exhale. Use your breathing like a boat would an anchor; it's something you can focus on whenever you begin feeling pain or stress.

Square breathing and box breathing are two of my favorite techniques—check out the steps below to try them!

Square breathing	Breathing Technique: 4-7-8
Square Breathing — Hold (1 2 3 4), Inhale (4 3 2 1 down), Exhale (1 2 3 4 down), Hold (4 3 2 1)	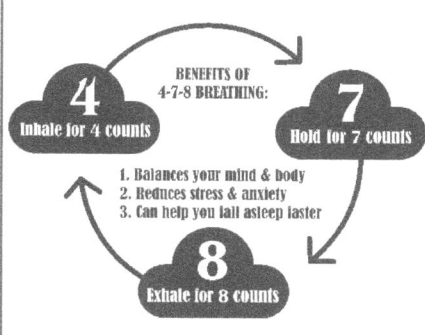 BENEFITS OF 4-7-8 BREATHING: 1. Balances your mind & body 2. Reduces stress & anxiety 3. Can help you fall asleep faster
1. Find a comfortable position, sitting on a chair or on the floor 2. Gently close your eyes. 3. Take a few deep breaths to prepare yourself for the practice. 4. Inhale for 4 seconds: Count 1…2…3…4 5. Hold that breath for 4 seconds: Count 1…2…3…4 6. Exhale for 4 seconds: Count 1…2…3…4 7. Hold again for another 4 seconds: Count 1…2…3…4 8. Repeat.	1. Find a comfortable position. Ensure you're in a safe and quiet space. 2. Gently close your eyes. Prepare for your breathing practice and take a few deep breaths. 3. Inhale for 4 seconds: Count 1…2…3…4 4. Hold your breath for 7 seconds: Count 1…2…3…4…5…6…7 5. Exhale for 8 seconds: Count 1…2…3…4…5…6…7…8

Mindful breathing harnesses your body's natural processes, resulting in the relief of RA symptoms. It's a free way to relieve pain, inflammation, and stress!

I recommend continuing any breathing technique for at least five rounds. Over time, gradually extend the time you're consciously breathing to reach five or ten minutes. Do this practice twice daily for two weeks. After those two weeks, take a step back and reassess your progress.

Aim to answer these questions mentally:

- How do I feel?
- How is my pain? Has it improved?
- How is my anxiety?

Start writing down these in your diary, and every month, reassess the progress.

> **My advice on breathing techniques**
>
> Breathing practices might be difficult in the beginning. If you can't hold your breath for six or eight seconds, that's perfectly fine. Be gentle to yourself. Like meditation or mindfulness, breathing is a practice; it doesn't have to be perfect. With continued sessions, you'll be able to breathe like *a pro* with little effort in just a few weeks.

Shift Your Mindset: Healthy Stress-Reduction Practices

Meditation and mindfulness are relatively broad, overarching habits that, while beneficial, can feel a little intangible to beginners. While both are relatively easy to integrate, fully embracing them is difficult for those without experience in either practice.

Luckily for my patients who feel a little apprehensive about these, there are a few other, more "*beginner-friendly*" tools you can try and use to start a healthier, more stress-free lifestyle. Don't jump into the deep end—start your mindfulness and healthy mindset journey with these smaller, perhaps more straightforward tools like quitting complaining, starting a gratitude journal, or even learning about savoring the moments.

Quit the Complaining Habit

We complain at least once a minute on average during any typical conversation. That's a lot—way more than most of us intend to.

Complaining is formed just like any other habit. When we complain, the neurons in our brains connect, creating bridges. As a result, our brains tell us to repeat the action, hence why we don't even notice we're complaining in the first place!

Complaining and negativity are holding you back. Researchers at Stanford University recently found that complaining causes structural changes in our brains and shrinks the hippocampus, the part of our brain connected to problem-solving and conscious thought. Additionally, complaining causes the body to release more cortisol—the stress hormone. As we discussed in earlier chapters, cortisol shifts your body and mind into fight or flight mode, raising your blood pressure and blood sugar and diminishing your immune system's functioning, a cause for concern for those struggling with RA.

In contrast, simply thinking positive thoughts or counting the positive things in your life and savoring them can make you feel happier and improve your overall health.[20]

What's the solution? There are many!

Firstly, surrounding ourselves with positive people can be a powerful way to mitigate complaining: Our brains naturally and unconsciously mimic the moods and words of those around us. Be cautious about spending your precious time with those who only complain; feel free to distance yourself if necessary.

Just like overeating, smoking, or drinking to excess, complaining isn't serving you or your disease. Complaining impairs your immune system function and raises your blood pressure, causing more inflammation and pain. In contrast, positivity helps reduce pain and improves overall health.

Stop complaining and replace the habit with a more positive attitude! Not only will you feel happier, but symptom improvement will follow.

How to stop complaining?

1. **When you complain, ensure there's a clear purpose.**
   a. What are you looking for when you complain?
   b. What's the purpose of the complaint?
   c. What's your goal?
2. **Start with something positive.** Before complaining, use a positive phrase or statement. Try to counteract the complaint.
3. **Be specific.** Identify just one reason why you're complaining and describe that reason. Don't regale those around you with the whole situation. Pinpoint what's wrong.
4. **End with a positive attitude.** If you want a resolution to your problem, be kind. Show that you're hopeful this situation has a happy ending.

Say "Thank You": Gratitude and RA

Waking up with RA-related pain in your mind isn't easy. The good news is that we can rewire parts of the brain responsible for pain to bring it down to a more manageable level.

Gratitude is one method used to do this: Gratitude is a positive emotion you can cultivate yourself. It involves recognizing and appreciating what you've received in life. Furthermore, it has recently emerged as a potential pain and stress-management tactic.

You might've heard of gratitude journaling already: Gratitude journaling has grown in popularity recently. I highly recommend it to boost and cultivate the gratitude you feel with and in your life.

Skeptics might find this a little silly, but journaling about the positive things in your life is a vital skill and resource. Research shows that taking conscious time to experience gratitude makes you feel happier and can positively affect your overall health.[21] In other words, *thinking about* what you're grateful for yields greater happiness.

Additionally, studies show that *writing about* these enhances happiness and improves our coping ability. Gratitude also yields better mood, higher energy levels, and less anxiety. In the context of pain, particularly pain from RA, this is a powerful realization—journaling about the positive and negative things in your life can help you understand your pain, alleviating it by taking away its power over your mood.

What are the health benefits of gratitude?
- Improves heart health
- Lowers anxiety and depression
- Improves sleep
- Lower perception of pain

Gratitude journaling is much like other kinds of journaling—you need yourself, a writing tool, and a piece of paper or notebook. I recommend purchasing a notebook specifically for gratitude journaling and keeping your records in one place. You're welcome to use my *Rheumatoid arthritis Journal, which I designed specifically* for patients like you. Check the resource section for more information and a link to this.

> **○ PROTIP**
>
> **Every day,** *think and write down* **three things you are grateful for.**

Write down three things you're grateful for each day, and be specific. These don't need to be significant realizations, and small things are perfectly acceptable, particularly when you don't feel very grateful. For example, you might write, "I'm grateful for my morning cup of tea," or, "I'm grateful for the kind lady at the checkout counter in the grocery store."

You can also cultivate gratitude by expressing it to another person: One of my favorite tips is to write another person a gratitude letter. Research shows that this practice dramatically impacts your happiness and the person receiving the letter, yielding an overall positive outcome.

> **Bonus tip: not-so random acts of kindness**
>
> Happy people are motivated to do kind things for others: Studies show that engaging in kind acts boosts your mood and sense of social connection. For the next week, aim to perform a daily act of kindness beyond what you might normally do for another person. These don't have to be over-the-top or time-intensive acts, but they should be something that helps or impacts another person or group of people. Write down your random act of kindness in your notebook at the end of each day.

Live in the Happy Moments

Often, we fail to stay in the moment and let our minds wander to think about connotations, responsibilities, and expectations; because of this, we don't truly allow ourselves to enjoy what's in front of us.

Savoring is briefly stepping outside of an experience to review and appreciate it. It intensifies and prolongs the positive emotions that accompany doing something, being around someone, or engaging in the things we love.

A few years ago, researchers looked at the benefits of savoring one's ability to react positively to the events that come their way, and on overall happiness.[22] Daily savoring helped over 100 participants more positively relate to those around them and boosted the number of happy or positive events they experienced, demonstrating that savoring powerfully benefits your mindset.

Improving our mindfulness and meditation practices can help with savoring: These practices help us pay attention to and understand what's going on directly in front of us, which, in turn, allows us to notice the good along with the bad.

> **How can you practice savoring?**
>
> 1. **Share your experiences with another person.** Ensure this person is someone you enjoy, and the savoring will happen naturally.
> 2. **Unplug your electronics.** Enjoy your time free from unnecessary distractions. Block out this time, and stick to it.
> 3. **Consider yourself lucky.** Imagine how lucky you are to enjoy that moment when you're genuinely enjoying something.
> 4. **Each night, note in a journal why you savored something that day.** Look back at that list as often as you need to, and be sure to repeat those activities in the future.

For the next week, practice savoring: Pick one experience you wish to savor daily. You might pick a nice hot shower, a delicious meal, your morning walk, or anything, as long as you genuinely enjoy it. Similar to gratitude journaling, note what you savored each night. Review what you've savored on previous days to help motivate you.

Savoring is a gift you give yourself. The practice helps cultivate positivity and a healthy mindset, paving the way for lower stress and pain levels. Give it a try today!

Your Stress-Free Journey

RA is stressful—that much is true. Patients are stuck navigating uncomfortable, and sometimes unrelenting pain and discomfort, not to mention arduous schedules full of treatments and doctor visits. All of this is inherently stressful, but as we've discussed throughout this chapter, stress isn't serving you, and it indeed isn't serving your RA.

Stress aggravates symptoms through interactions with the nervous system and increased cortisol levels. Unfortunately, these interactions yield more pain, inflammation, and more swelling. In this Chapter, we focused on techniques to reduce stress and RA-related pain. We examined the benefits of mindfulness and meditation, which reduce discomfort and boost mood. Then, we touched on breathing techniques and how breathing impacts inflammation. Finally, we discussed some simple tools, like gratitude and savoring, to help you take stress-reduction step by step.

Reduce your stress and unlock a life free from pesky symptoms! Use the tools and tips we discussed in this chapter to cut your stress levels and regain your perspective. I assure you—you can make these simple changes. All it takes is knowledge and just a few minutes of your time.

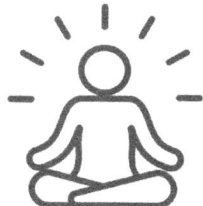

CHAPTER 8

MOTION IS LOTION: HOW TO GET MOVIN'

The correlation between exercise and your health is well-documented, and for good reason. Our bodies are designed to move; without movement, our bodies and joints become stale. I always tell my patients that the opposite of *"motion is lotion"* is *"when you rest, you rust."* Motion is lotion for your body and, most notably for those struggling with RA, your joints.

Exercise has been associated with excellent health for thousands of years. Unfortunately, in our modern landscape, exercise has become more challenging. Thousands of years ago, we couldn't rely on cars, buses, subways, or bikes to take us where we needed to go. Instead, we used our own two feet for transportation. Today, many people only move from one transportation mode to another: from their house to their car, their car to an elevator, and their elevator to their workspace. As you read this chapter, challenge yourself to think of a few ways to start prioritizing movement in your daily life.

What Are The Benefits of Exercise?

Exercise means movement, which can be anything from taking the stairs to going on a morning walk or prioritizing standing while at work. Like nutritious food, exercise gives your body the strength and fuel to do everything you do in a day—even the small stuff.

But why do it? Studies show that exercise has a similar mood-boosting effect to antidepressants and improves your longevity.[1,2] Furthermore, a lack of exercise plays a role in the development of multiple chronic conditions, including heart disease, diabetes, high blood pressure, and certain types of cancer (including liver, breast, colorectal, and lung cancer).[3]

Exercise provides you and your body with many benefits—check out the box for a summary.

Benefits of exercise on health

- Maintains normal weight
- Improves bone density and muscle mass
- Lessens your risk of chronic diseases
- Relieves stress
- Improves memory and cognition
- Improves sleep quality
- Lessens anxiety and depression symptoms
- Improves your sex life

Exercise & RA: Motion is Lotion For Your Joints

You might assume that beginning an exercise regimen when you have a lot of swelling and joint pain would be damaging to your suffering joints. But is this true?

When you wake up with a lot of stiffness, you might notice that stretching and moving are helping—right?

Then, should you exercise or should you not?

Many of my patients ask this question, and my answer is loud and clear: "Yes, you should exercise!"

If you suffer from RA, you understand how common and devastating stiffness can be. Luckily, movement can prevent stiffness. This is where your joint's cartilage comes into play: Cartilage acts as a cushion between your bones. However, it doesn't have access to a direct blood supply. Instead, it relies solely on movement to deliver essential nutrients and oxygen to keep it healthy. Therefore, movement supports healthy joints, which, in turn, helps keep stiffness at bay!

Additionally, regular movement helps your body produce more synovial fluid, the lubricating fluid bathing our joints. As you see, *"motion is lotion"* is a common phrase in physical therapy because it's true!

> *The opposite of "motion is lotion" is*
> *"when you rest, you rust."*

Exercise also improves energy levels, lessens fatigue, improves pain, and plays a significant role in weight loss.[4-6] The evidence for RA patients is clear: A 2015 study found that exercise can improve inflammation, lessen heart disease risk, and improve mental health.[7] Other studies corroborate this: A systematic literature review examining exercise's benefits found that RA patients who engaged in any form of movement enjoyed lower disease activity, inflammation marker levels, fatigue, and improved joint function.[8] Exercise is beneficial even in elderly patients; in this population specifically, those who exercised for 20 weeks experienced a significant improvement in their overall health.[9]

So, here's my advice: Everyone with RA should exercise! Engaging in exercise alleviates some of the pain caused by your swollen joints, reduces inflammation, and decreases bone loss.

How to Get Movin'

After explaining the benefits of exercise, many patients ask me, "What exercises should you try?"

"Are some better than others?"

"Is there an optimal time to move?"

In this section, we'll cover everything you need to know to get started with exercise!

Experts, including myself, know that RA patients benefit significantly from moderate-intensity exercises. Studies show that this helps reduce fatigue and address many of the most common concerns I hear in my office, like pain, stiffness, and persistent swelling.

Within the realm of moderate-intensity exercises, you have plenty of options. I encourage patients to find movements for their unique symptoms and needs. For example, a woman suffering from a mild form of RA who used to be a dance instructor might enjoy and benefit from twice-weekly Zumba classes and morning yoga. On the other hand, this could be out of reach for an older patient who comes to me with little exercise history or athletic ability. In that case, I recommend morning stretching and daily 30-minute walks.

> Find exercises you enjoy that fit within your busy lifestyle. See how you respond to a particular movement pattern, then incorporate the exercises that work best for your symptoms and your life.

After discussing *how* patients should exercise, many ask about *when*. While there's no "right time" to exercise, many patients report that moving in the morning—often first thing—is the best way to stave off painful aches later in the day. This practice curbs their morning stiffness.

Begin your day with gentle stretching exercises (check out the next section and the resource chapter at the end of the book for some examples). As you start feeling better and your disease is better controlled, you can incorporate more vigorous exercises into your routine, like jogging, dancing, or an exercise class.

> **Where should I exercise?**
>
> The best place to exercise is where you feel good about doing so: This might be at your home, the gym, or in a class setting.

PRACTICAL ADVICE

- Before beginning an exercise regimen, take the following steps:
- Choose an exercise that's fun and convenient for you.
- Make realistic short and long-term goals for yourself.
- Identify the obstacles likely to keep you from exercising (children, morning routine, fatigue, etc.) and devise a plan to overcome them before trying an exercise program.
- Find a friend or family member to exercise with—they can help keep you accountable.
- Keep a log of your exercises on a calendar and give yourself small rewards as you keep to the schedule you crafted.

Cori Gramescu is an internationally acclaimed fitness trainer who was kind enough to demonstrate a few essential exercises for you (See the pictures below). With Dr. Melissa Koehl, a physical therapist specializing in arthritis, I've developed a program available for my patients, but you may also find it in my online course. Both of these experts offer years of experience working with arthritis patients. On my YouTube channel, you'll find free videos illustrating different forms of exercise, including yoga, for patients with RA. For now, check out the exercises below to start your movement journey.

Cat Cow Pose

Start on your hands and knees. Round your back toward the ceiling while dropping your head and tucking your rear end. Return to the middle, arch your back, and lift your head. This pose can improve spinal mobility and alleviate low back pain. Note: You can also incorporate breathing into this exercise–inhale as you round your back, exhale as your arch your back. Repeat 4-6 times.

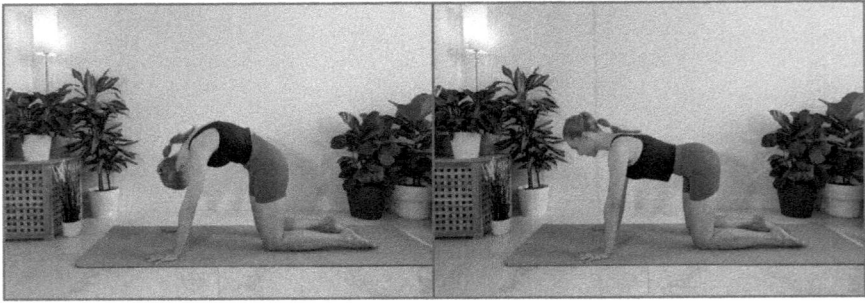

Chair Pose

Stand with your feet apart. Raise your arms and take a deep breath. Next, lower your arms halfway and squat as if you were going to sit in a chair (exhale as you squat). This pose can strengthen your legs and improve balance. Repeat 4-6 times.

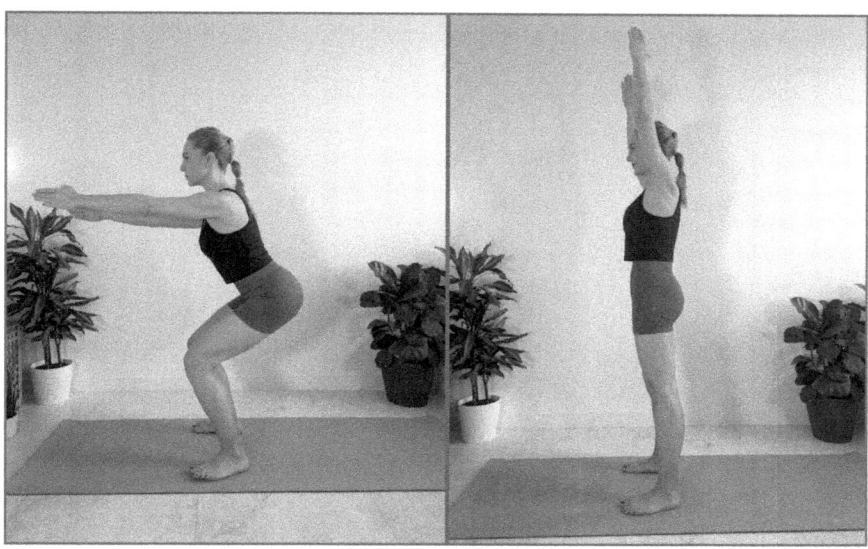

Forward Fold

Stand with your knees bent slightly, inhale deeply. Bend forward while exhaling and let your arms hang. This gentle stretch can alleviate tension in the back and hamstrings. Repeat 4-6 times.

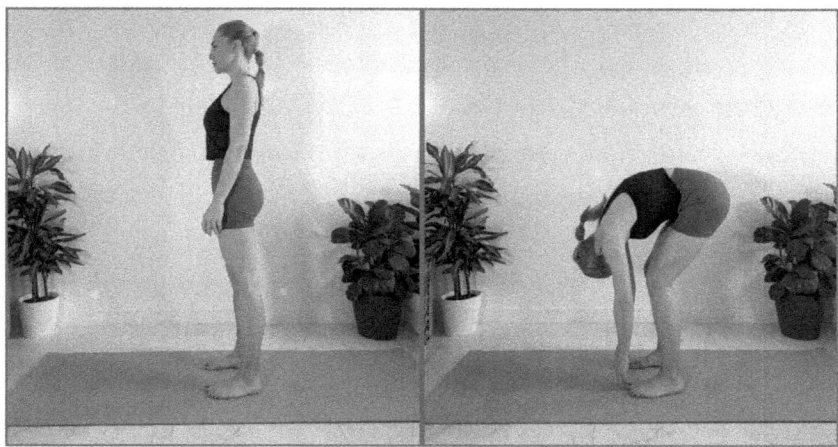

Side Angle Pose

Stand with your feet about 4 feet apart. Turn your right foot out to a 90-degree angle and the other to about 45 degrees. Inhale deeply. Exhale as you bend your right knee and bring your elbow to rest on it while your other arm extends over your head. Come back to the middle and repeat on the other side. This pose can improve balance and strength. Repeat 4 times on each side, being careful to position your foot each time.

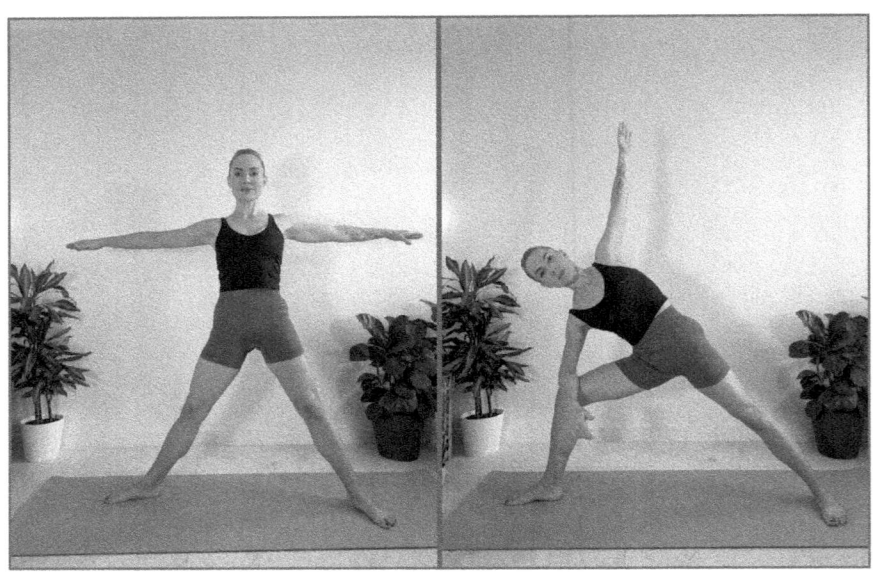

Aquatic Therapy

Joan was 60-years-old when she started experiencing joint pain, swelling, and stiffness in her wrists and knees. Initially, she thought that these were related to aging, but when she couldn't get out of bed one morning, she realized that her symptoms might be indicative of something else.

When Joan came to my office, she was in tears. Before her diagnosis, Joan was very active, and enjoyed walking in the park, playing tennis, and Zumba class with her friends; her inability to engage in these activities felt insurmountable to her.

Together, we walked through the steps of diagnosis, and I diagnosed her with RA. Joan began treatment and nearly returned to her old self in six months. However, when she tried to go back to her previous activities, she couldn't handle the pain. RA had left her endurance much decreased.

When Joan returned to see me for a follow-up visit, she asked, "What do I do? Every time I try to exercise, I'm in pain the next day!"

"Joan, I have some advice for you," I told her. "Have you ever thought about doing some water exercises?"

"No—tell me more," she replied. "I have a pool at home that I could use."

"Sure," I said, nodding. "You can use your pool at home or check out some therapy pools in your area—the water in those is warmer, about 91-92 degrees Fahrenheit. There are also some local classes specifically designed for people with arthritis."

Joan nodded at me, and I continued, "The water takes some of the gravitational pressure off your body, which means less stress on your joints. It might help you build up your stamina again."

I handed her a pamphlet showcasing some local classes. "Why not give it a try?" she said.

She began attending classes at a local pool, where they taught water exercise. When she came back a few weeks later, she told me that the first time she got in, she felt like she was floating: The water held her up, and she didn't feel the pain she'd felt before when she tried to get back into exercising. The warm water relaxed her muscles, and with every movement, she felt supported.

"I barely feel any pain anymore!" she said happily after a few months. "My swelling has nearly disappeared, and I finally feel like myself again." At that moment, I couldn't have been happier for her.

Water exercise, also known as Aquatic therapy, or hydrotherapy, is a low-impact activity that's highly valuable to patients with RA, like Joan. It can help improve circulation, ease pain and anxiety, and promote relaxation. One study found that aquatic therapy, when combined with medication, eased joint RA patients' pain and tenderness more than medication alone.[10]

Aquatic therapy has been proven to be a more effective intervention for RA patients compared to out-of-the-water exercises like jogging, yoga, or biking. Another scientific study found that patients who engaged in hydrotherapy were more likely to feel much better physically and mentally than those who exercised out of water.[11] Furthermore, a systematic review illustrated aquatic therapy's positive impact on patient's pain, joint tenderness, mood, and grip strength compared to those who exercised traditionally or not at all.[12]

Many local or public pools offer free or reduced-cost membership, and don't be afraid to ask around for a friend or family member who might have a backyard swimming area! Also, this *is* a good time to Google and look up arthritis exercise programs in your area. Many of them offer aquatic therapy programs tailored to arthritis patients!

Keep On Movin'

While there's no right way to exercise or move more, there *is* a wrong way! Not exercising or foregoing exercise or movement can have severe consequences. Without daily movement and regular exercises, you can't benefit from the scope of benefits exercise provides, including reduced pain, improved function and mood, and less joint pain and stiffness.

Check out the resource section of this book for more information, and look at my online course, which includes more than 80 exercises designed to address the needs of people with all forms of RA.

I recommend that all of my patients and everyone move a little more throughout the day. Not only will you thank me, but your joints will thank you.

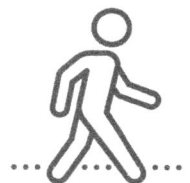

CHAPTER

9

GET SOME REST: SLEEP & RA

Did you know the average person spends about a third of their life asleep? That's more time than we spend with family and, for some of us, even working. Since we do it so often, it must be important. In this chapter, we'll discuss sleep's vital role in our health and well-being, our bodily processes, and the relationship between sleep and RA.

What Is Sleep?

Just like your phone or laptop needs to recharge, so do you. Sleep is a physiological need—the essential mechanism by which our body recharges.

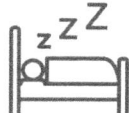

> *Why We Sleep* by Dr. Matthew Walker, expert sleep researcher, and scientist, discusses sleep's transformative power and how we can harness it to improve our health. *Why We Sleep* changed how I thought about and understood sleep, and I highly recommend it.

You might not know it, but your body is busy while you're sleeping. Here's a summary of all of the things your body is so busy doing while you get a little shut-eye:

- Lowers your heart rate and blood pressure, promoting relaxation
- Produces and regulates hormones like estrogen, testosterone, and leptin, the hormone that regulates hunger
- Prepares your liver to absorb fats properly
- Restores healthy insulin levels
- Forms and stores memories
- Boosts your immune system, ensuring it's ready to fight disease and infections
- Regulates and restores emotional balance

Do you remember when you were young and bragging about sleeping just a few hours a night? Maybe you were at a sleepover, and you and your friends wanted to see who could stay up the longest. What we didn't know then was how important sleep truly is.

> **Did you know?**
> Staying awake for more than sixteen hours straight decreases your cognitive abilities and performance as much as two glasses of wine.

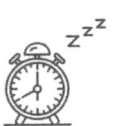

Sleep is as essential to our health as a trip to the doctor, and those who don't receive enough of it or enough quality sleep can suffer serious consequences. I can't stress enough how crucial sleep is to your health. We can't just have enough of it; we also need high-quality sleep to function correctly. In other words, the body needs ample sleep time to do what it needs to do to be you!

Short-term vs long-term consequences of poor sleep	
Short-term consequences	Long-term consequences
• Brain fog • Fatigue • Poor focus and attention • Pain	• Heart disease • Diabetes • Infertility • Mood disorders • Hypertension • Obesity • Stroke • Alzheimer's disease • Lower immune system

Often, we prioritize work, school, responsibilities, and chores above sleep, leaving us feeling less productive instead of more. We might think that sacrificing a few hours of sleep isn't a big deal, but it is. Humans are the only mammals who knowingly delay sleep and, thus, suffer the consequences: Research shows that sacrificing your sleep, even just for one night causes decreased efficiency and effectiveness for days beyond the night you decided to stay up a little too late.[2]

Sleep doesn't equate to laziness. In fact, it boosts productivity, cognition, and our ability to form memories.

Why Is Sleep So Important For Those With RA?

When Amanda was referred to my practice, she was 40 years old. After she had her first baby at 38, Amanda began noticing tingling and numbness in her hands while she rocked and held her baby, which made breastfeeding difficult. Initially, she thought that the pain was related to carpal tunnel syndrome and knew that, because she'd just had a baby, this was common.

As her symptoms grew worse, so did their effect on her ability to care for her child. Amanda sought the help of her PCP, who referred her to a hand surgeon. The surgeon noticed the pronounced swelling in both of her hands and referred her to my office.

During my intake session with Amanda, she told me that she'd seen some signs of swelling, pain, tingling, and numbness toward the end of her pregnancy. The symptoms seemed to subside after a week or two, so she didn't think anything of them. Unfortunately, the symptoms worsened to an unmanageable level about a few months after she gave birth, and since then, she'd been experiencing them nearly daily.

After a few tests, I diagnosed Amanda with RA. We promptly started treatment, but three months later, she came back to me for a follow-up in tears.

"I can't do this anymore," she cried, burying her face in her hands. "I'm still in so much pain—nothing seems to work. What am I doing wrong?" she asked me.

"You're doing nothing wrong, Amanda," I told her. I felt my heart pang, and I began to think.

"Tell me about your baby," I said, trying to understand the situation more deeply.

Amanda's face lit up when she told me about her baby boy, who was now nearly a toddler. "He loves trouble," she said, laughing. "And he *hates* to sleep."

I nodded and began to understand the situation Amanda was in. She was unable to sleep during the day due to her work, and her baby's crying kept her up incessantly at night. She was receiving less than five hours of sleep, which aggravated her pain.

"I think sleep is the issue here," I explained. "Why do you think we need to sleep?" She was confused and intrigued, and I began to explain to Amanda the role of sleep for our health, the connection with her fatigue, and the impact of chronic sleep deprivation on her pain.

After five or so months, and with some help from her partner, she changed her sleep habits and could finally sleep for 7-8 hours every night. Her fatigue and pain improved, and she was more productive and focused.

Like Amanda, over 60% of RA patients report poor sleep quality and quantity, averaging only 5.7 hours per night, new baby or not. Furthermore,

RA patients tend to experience fragmented sleep that aggravates their pain sensitivity the day following.

> ○ **PROTIP**
>
> **Aim to sleep 8-9 hours each night. Sleeping better will decrease your pain.**

Sleep plays an integral role in regulating the immune system: When you sleep, bodily processes calm your immune response, thus lessening inflammation.[3] In RA patients, poor sleep quality and insomnia can cause excessive inflammation, and vice versa; excessive inflammation and more pain lessen sleep quality.

The two—sleep and pain–exist in a *bidirectional relationship* with one another, with poorer sleep causing more pain and more pain, in turn, causing poorer sleep. Studies corroborate this: One study found that poor sleep quality (or little sleep) caused an uptick in RA patients' disease activity, pain, physical and mental health, and fatigue.[4]

Other studies show similar, reciprocal findings: RA patients with higher disease activity are more likely to experience[5]

- insomnia
- poor sleep quality
- poor mental health, and
- lessened cognitive responses.

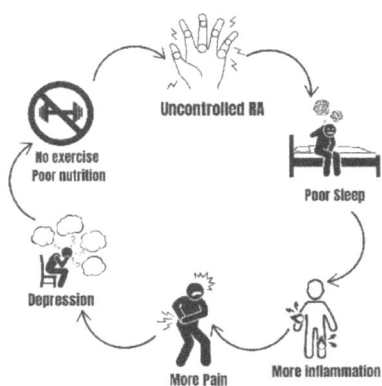

Figure 5. The relationship between sleep, pain and Rheumatoid arthritis

Luckily, getting more sleep and taking steps can mitigate your pain, thus improving your sleep. Studies point to sleep playing an essential role in a person's physical well-being: RA patients who sleep more and have better sleep quality enjoy a higher quality of life.[6]

How Can You Improve Your Sleep?

We've established that poor sleep aggravates pain, and more pain worsens sleep. But how can we break this vicious cycle? It's up to you to make sleep a top priority. Use the techniques you learned in the previous chapters, like breathing, mindfulness, and meditation (and learn about others, like guided imagery or body scanning), to help you sleep better.

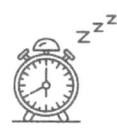

Here are a few pieces of practical advice that I share with my patients to help them achieve more restful sleep:

1. **Begin waking up at the same time each day.** This isn't easy—I know this firsthand. Many tend to sleep less on weekdays, catching up on lost sleep on weekends, but this only confuses our bodies. This practice is called "*social jet lag.*"

   Think about time zones; when you experience social jet lag, your brain lives in two different time zones, and these lags disrupt your sleep routine. Maintain a balanced sleep routine on both weekends and weekdays. Teach your brain to respect your routine and to support your sleep.

2. **Go to sleep when you feel sleepy.** This tip might seem simple, but it's true. Many of us ignore sleepiness, choosing instead to engage in an activity, like answering emails, that isn't conducive to rest. As with exercise, listen to your body and the signals it's sending you.

3. **Eat a relatively early light dinner (around 6 pm).** Late-night gorging and snacking are disastrous for your diet and even more so for your sleep. If your body is busy digesting a large meal, it's not focusing on propelling you into the restful and restorative stages of sleep you need to be your best self.

4. **Set a low temperature in your bedroom (about 65 F or 18 C degrees).** Your body temperature follows your circadian rhythm, and so does your

sleep cycle. You feel sleepiest when your body temperature is low and most awake when your body temperature is high.

Ensure the temperature in your space is *cool* but *not cold*.

5. **Your bedroom is for sleep and intimacy, not for meetings or movies.** Try your best to manage and balance your space accordingly. Don't answer emails, watch the news, or turn on a fast-paced action movie before sleep; designate your room as a space for sleep and intimacy.

   Keep the room where you sleep dark and quiet, and feel free to use a sleep mask to keep excess light out. Mentally, this helps your brain associate your sleep space with relaxation, not work.

6. **Make sleep a routine and stick to it.** Dim all of the lights in your home 30 minutes before bedtime. Listen to soothing music or engage in an activity that relaxes you, like sipping a lukewarm mug of tea or reading a book. Wind down, and your body will, too.

   You can't jump in bed and expect to fall asleep immediately. Your mind and body won't simply shut off after a busy day—you're not a light switch! Give yourself about an hour before bed, and use this hour to perform your bedtime routine, read, or do some mindful meditation. Practice techniques like mindful breathing or body scanning to get your brain in a place to rest.

7. **Unplug:** Eliminate technology from your nighttime routine. Devices such as your mobile phone, tablet or computer emit blue light, which can interfere with melanin production, which is responsible for regulating your sleep-wake cycle. This can make it more difficult for you to fall asleep naturally.

   If you want to set an alarm, put the clock or phone out of sight but close enough to hear it when it rings in the morning.

8. **Avoid exercise and alcohol two to three hours before bedtime.** Alcohol reduces the amount of restorative deep sleep you get overnight and can cause you to wake up throughout your sleep cycle.

   Exercise is a vigorous activity that doesn't align with the restful environment you've created. Avoid it before bedtime, and exercise earlier in the day.

9. **Be consistent in your routine.** Stick to it, even on weekends, once you've established a routine that works for you. Aim for between *seven and nine hours of sleep* daily—this is the recommended amount for most adults.

Get Started With Better Sleep

In short, sleep has many benefits. Not only does sleep improve a patient's mood and lessen pain and inflammation, but it also prepares you to take on the next day! Use the information in the chapter to improve your sleep and escape the vicious cycle of sleeplessness and pain.

The tips I've provided in this chapter are among my favorites, but you can try plenty of sleep hacks—check out my website (linked in the resource section) for more information about healthy sleep and tips to boost your rest.

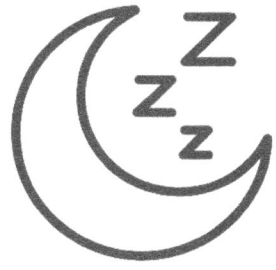

CHAPTER 10

NATURAL REMEDIES THAT WORK (AND THOSE THAT DON'T)

Susan was a long-time patient, and she was frustrated when she came into my office. Despite years of working together, traditional treatments didn't seem to work well for Susan: We'd cycled through nearly all of the tools in my toolbox, and still, she was in pain.

Susan looked a little guilty at this appointment, hiding her face with her hands. "Are you okay?" I asked, eager to understand what she was going through.

"You're gonna be upset," she replied, and I chuckled. "I tried this fish tank therapy I saw on social media. Everyone online said it worked wonders for people with RA pain, and I thought it couldn't hurt."

I was instantly concerned. "What happened?"

"Well," she paused, taking off her shoes. "It didn't help with my pain at all, and now I have this redness I can't get rid of."

I examined Susan's feet, her usual area of concern. Each was bright red and swollen, not from RA, but from what looked like an infection.

"Is it bad?" she asked, apprehensive to look.

"We need to get you on antibiotics as soon as possible," I said, concerned but deliberately careful. I've heard of fish tank therapy causing infections, and I think that's what's happening here."

Luckily, Susan's infection cleared up after a few weeks, but I knew, and she learned, that the situation could've become more severe.

At her follow-up, she was nearly healed. "I won't make that mistake again," she laughed.

I nodded, "It's okay to Google, but you can't try everything you see or hear online."

As you've learned, and as Susan realized that day, there's a lot of "fake news" surrounding RA, the symptoms it causes, and, even worse, how to treat it naturally.

A few times in this book, I've mentioned how Googling certain components of RA (including the disease, treatment, and foods that are "good" for RA) can yield negative results. Now, for the purposes of a short exercise, I invite you to Google an RA-related question you've been dwelling on lately. Your question can be anything, as long as it's RA-related. What comes up when you do this?

When I did this exercise, I Googled "natural treatments for RA." The first few links on my page were sponsored advertisements from prescription companies and a handful of articles published by relatively reputable publications. Scrolling down my page were 8 advertisements for books about RA, but only one was published by a doctor or physician. Below that were links to discussion forums and more advertisements for 'natural' creams and pills that claim to help RA-related symptoms.

So, beyond a few somewhat reputable sites, all I got were ads! Written using language meant to invite you to click on the drug or tool, advertisements are designed to garner your attention quickly. Moreso, the bright colors and promises used by these advertisements are meant to do one thing and one thing only—they're meant to make you buy the product, pill, or service they're selling.

Advertisers and marketing agencies manipulate your pain, turning it into a money-making tool: They know that RA is painful and exhausting, so they showcase happy, smiling people moving around freely. For most, this isn't the reality. Few RA patients realistically feel this way, and even with treatment, only 60-70% of patients feel notably better. Advertisers are savvy and understand that your pain and exhaustion will cause you to look for natural alternatives. Many advertised natural remedies are backed by minimal if any, scientific proof. Besides not helping improve symptoms, these may hurt you. Unfortunately, many patients buy into the promises made by marketers because they think "natural" means "safe". Advertisers make millions of dollars a year selling false promises, profiting off your pain.

Wouldn't you rather listen to a doctor with over twenty years of academic and professional experience treating your condition, telling you that this specific medication will work as opposed to a marketer whose job is to profit off of your pain? I certainly would!

Often, patients come into my office having Googled a few of these and, while sitting on my exam table, ask, "So—does X, Y, or Z really work?" Then, I'm tasked with explaining to them which "natural remedies" potentially help based on the scientific evidence we have so far, and which remedies do not.

In this section, we'll discuss more so-called "natural remedies" and clarify whether they can potentially help fall flat–or worse yet, cause harm. My goal is for you to avoid spending excess money and keep your safe and healthy.

Natural Remedies That Don't Work

Many patients find traditional RA treatments (check out Chapter 3 for more details) a little scary and are inclined to test more "natural" or "holistic" alternatives. I completely understand this. In fact, as a physician, I aim to bridge two worlds: western medicine and a more holistic, natural approach.

Unfortunately, though advertised as "better" alternatives, natural remedies often have little scientific evidence backing them up. Think about Susan's case! Although fish tank therapy was advertised as helping decrease inflammation, it did nothing to help her symptoms and caused a severe foot infection. This is UNSAFE! So, when patients come into my office asking if these natural products, X, Y, or Z, will work for them, I base my recommendations on the scientific evidence I find.

Let's dive deeper and discuss commonly advertised options to treat RA!

Magnet Therapy

Some people believe that magnets can influence blood flow and iron, delivering essential nutrients to your joints and thus, alleviating some of the pain and inflammation. While I'd love to believe this, I must tell you that this theory is a myth.

The iron in our blood isn't ferromagnetic, meaning it's not attracted to the pull of a magnet. No scientific evidence indicates that magnets, whether in free, bracelet, or sticker form, alter blood flow.[1]

Think about what happens when you do an MRI: If this theory were valid, all of the iron in your body would be pulled toward the machine, causing you to explode. This doesn't happen, and the few studies that examine magnet therapy show that it's not an effective intervention for those with RA.

Copper Bracelets

Copper bracelets are promoted as a potential remedy for RA because of copper's presumed anti-inflammatory properties. This recommendation is based on misguided science: While some evidence indicates that those deficient in copper develop more inflammation, copper can't be absorbed effectively through the skin, so those wearing copper bracelets won't experience any benefits to their

RA pain or inflammation. In other words, bracelets can improve your appearance or go with your outfit as jewelry, but they won't help your RA.²

Fish Tank Therapy

Fish tank therapy involves immersing your feet or hands into a tank of small fish that nibble away dead skin and improve RA symptoms. While there are some anecdotal stories from those who report improvement, I think this therapy is ludicrous: There's no scientific evidence supporting the idea that a fish tank will benefit you or your RA symptoms.

Fish tank therapy can cause infection through a bacteria called Mycobacterium avium. This bacteria can cause a severe infection for RA patients on immunosuppressive drugs. In short, it can cause much more harm than good.

Ozone Therapy

Ozone is a colorless gas made up of three oxygen atoms, and ozone therapy  involves introducing medical-grade ozone into the body. Those undergoing this therapy use ozone intravenously, through insufflation in the rectum or vagina, or through injection into the tissue.

Some believe that ozone therapy decreases inflammation, pain, and disease activity in people with RA. While it's been proven minimally effective at reducing inflammation in mice, no concrete clinical data suggest this therapy is effective in humans.³

Cherry Juice

Cherry juice contains flavonoids that have anti-inflammatory and antioxidant properties, which is why some propose that it might be beneficial for those struggling with RA.⁴

While cherry juice may contain these anti-inflammatory compounds, today's evidence is limited to patients suffering from gout, not RA. So, as of now, the jury is out on its effectiveness.

Glucosamine and Collagen Supplements

Glucosamine and collagen supplements are promoted on the market for their benefits to patients' joints, particularly those suffering from osteoarthritis or *wear and tear* arthritis.

However, remember that there are multiple forms of arthritis, and RA is an autoimmune disease; its cause differs drastically from osteoarthritis. Some research shows the effectiveness of glucosamine, vitamin E, and collagen on mice and rats, but there's no clinical evidence of these supplements on humans struggling with RA.[5]

Bee Venom

Fly like a butterfly; sting like a bee! Because some studies suggest that bee venom has anti-inflammatory and analgesic properties, people promote it to help decrease RA inflammation. Yes, a few studies are available that examine bee venom therapy injected through acupuncture! However, results yield inconclusive answers. Furthermore, a 2014 study illustrating its effectiveness (and thus popularizing the myth) used low-quality data, failing to show bee venom therapy's potential benefits for those with RA.[6]

Be cautious: Bee venom therapy can cause severe allergic reactions, particularly if you have a history of allergies to bee stings.

Natural remedies that have NO scientific back-up
• Magnet bracelets
• Cooper bracelets
• Bee venom
• Ozone therapy
• Glucosamine and chondroitin supplements
• Cherry juice

Just Say 'No' to Remedies That Don't Work

Everyone wants to embrace Mother Nature's benefits, but there's a reason why scientists conduct thorough research to back their hypotheses. As you've learned, magnets, copper bracelets, fish tank therapy, and certain supplements will not help RA symptoms. I want you to be safe, so I encourage you to discuss your options with your physician. Instead of investing in these options, save money for natural remedies that work! Let's find out which ones are proven to benefit your symptoms.

Natural Remedies That Work

Before we begin, I'd like to give you a little disclaimer: Consult your doctor before incorporating any new treatment into your RA regimen. While the following treatments have been proven effective for RA patients, some can potentially interact negatively with your traditional treatment plan. Your doctor can tell you which will work (or won't) for you.

With that in mind, it's time to discuss those natural remedies that work! The following treatments have all been proven in scientific settings to work for those struggling with RA. I recommend you give them a try!

Vagus Nerve Stimulation

In Chapter 7, we discussed the vagus nerve's role in bodily relaxation.

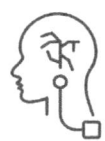

Moreover, in patients with RA, vagus nerve stimulation reduces pain and inflammation.[7] But how can we achieve this effect besides using breathing techniques? Simple! Newly designed devices send out electrical impulses that stimulate the vagus nerve. Some devices, like those that can be placed behind the ears for vagus nerve stimulation, are still in their testing phases. However, the results are quite promising, showing these devices are safe and help to improve disease activity in RA patients.[8]

How do you naturally stimulate the vagus nerve?
Square breathing
Laughing
Eating more fibers
Gargling with water
Singing loudly

Salt Baths

Adding salt to a bath, Epsom salt specifically, helps pain. Salt baths relax the muscles around your sore joints, sending signals through your nervous system to relax muscles and decrease pain levels. Studies examining RA patients support the use of salt baths and spas and show significant benefits in reducing the number of swollen and tender joints and, consequently, pain.[9]

Paraffin Wax Bath

If you had a recent manicure or pedicure, you were most likely offered a paraffin wax bath. You may think these are a great way to soothe rough skin, but did you know that paraffin wax relieves joint pain? This procedure particularly relieves pain and swelling in the small joints of your hands, which are frequently affected by RA.

I encourage my patients to use paraffin wax baths frequently, especially after a long day of activities in which they may overuse their hands (gardening, cleaning their house, or excessive typing). The warm paraffin wax relaxes your muscles, diminishing your stiffness and pain. Luckily, you don't need to go to an expensive spa or salon to get a paraffin wax treatment. You can buy a paraffin wax bath (which comes as a kit for the device and paraffin wax) from Amazon!

Manuka Honey

For centuries, honey has been used for its antibacterial and anti-inflammatory properties. Manuka honey, produced by bees pollinating tea trees in New Zealand and Australia, can help with bodily inflammation.[10] Manuka honey has been shown to reduce and regulate inflammatory cytokines produced by the body, thus reducing your RA symptoms. While your local grocery store might not carry it, Manuka honey is available online and at most health stores.

Warning: For those with diabetes, eat small quantities of manuka honey, as it can increase your blood sugar.

Melatonin

Many RA patients suffer from sleep disturbances and deprivation due to their chronic pain. As discussed in Chapter 9, less sleep aggravates pain, and more pain worsens sleep!

Melatonin is a hormone naturally produced in the body and regulates our sleep patterns. Some studies show that melatonin also yields anti-inflammatory properties, which is especially important for patients with RA.[11] Additionally, studies show that patients suffering from RA may have less melatonin in their bodies, which is correlated with higher disease activity, meaning more swollen and painful joints.[12]

Therefore, taking melatonin works twofold by improving your sleep quality, which reduces pain and improves your inflammation.

Sauna

Spending time in the sauna has been shown to improve blood circulation, 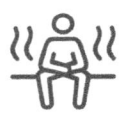 relax your muscles, reduce inflammation, and relieve pain. A sauna's heat and steam cause the body's muscles to relax and circulation to improve, which naturally improves swelling, stiffness, and fatigue, all common complaints of patients with RA.[13]

Infrared saunas are especially beneficial as their infrared waves penetrate deeply into your skin. Moreover, the heat from an infrared sauna releases endorphins—the body's feel-good chemicals—which interact with brain receptors, supporting feelings of happiness.[14] Better yet, endorphins yielded by time in the sauna reduce pain perception and enhance mood, making patients feel more relaxed.

CBD Oil or Cream

Many of my patients ask about CBD products (oil or cream), which are commonly advertised as a remedy for sleep, relaxation, pain, and inflammation. But do these really help?

Before we dive into the specifics of CBD (otherwise referred to as cannabidiol), let's lay the groundwork by discussing cannabis more broadly. Derived from the naturally flowering plant *Cannabis sativa*, cannabis harbors over 500 chemicals, including cannabinoids like tetrahydrocannabinol (THC), the primary psychoactive chemical in marijuana. However, unlike THC, CBD doesn't induce or cause any psychoactivity; according to the National Academies of Science, Engineering, and Medicine, "CBD is not impairing, meaning it does not cause you to feel 'high.'"[15]

CBD interacts with your body's cannabinoid receptors, namely the CB1 receptors on your nerves and joints and the CB2 receptors on your immune cells. These receptors and what "activates" them are pivotal in perceiving pain and how our immune system functions.

New evidence associates the cannabinoid system with rheumatic conditions like RA: It's believed that cannabis, and thus CBD, modulates the immune system.[16] CB2 activation decreases TNF-α levels (a molecule that induces inflammation), reducing oxidative stress and inflammation.[17] Furthermore, clinical studies confirm that CBD decreases levels of pro-inflammatory cytokines and influences how our T-cells interact, decreasing inflammation and, consequently, reducing pain.

> **What is the scientific evidence related to CBD?**
>
> Animal studies conducted at Dr. McDougall's Arthritis and Pain Lab in Canada showed that CBD:
> - Reduces pain levels
> - Repairs nerve damage
> - Lessens joint inflammation

The first study examining the use of cannabis-based medicine oil in patients with RA was conducted in 2006.[18] Researchers looked at over 50 RA patients, asking half to use Sativex (a combination of tetrahydrocannabinol (THC) and cannabidiol (CBD)) daily for five weeks. Patients who used this cannabis product experienced

- less pain
- less inflammation
- lower disease activity, and
- better sleep with minimal side effects.

More recent studies found the use of CBD oil reduces opiate use in arthritis patients, including those suffering from osteoarthritis, a common complication of long-term RA. CBD oil might also improve fatigue and sleep, two common complaints in RA patients.[16]

As a result of these vast benefits, CBD use has tripled over the past few years. In 2014, only 6% of RA patients used CBD oil for pain relief.[19] In 2019, about 18% of RA patients reported that they used CBD oil. 80% of these patients reported symptom relief.

In 2022, researchers created an anonymous questionnaire to evaluate CBD's efficacy in treating arthritis.[20] More than 400 patients, many with osteoarthritis and RA, responded. Interestingly, after using CBD oil or cream, about 60% of respondents reported using less medication (including anti-inflammatories, acetaminophen, and opioids). Approximately 20% of respondents stopped using anti-inflammatories and opioids entirely. Better yet, all these people reported improved pain, physical function, and sleep quality.

Recently, the National Arthritis Foundation conducted an online survey of over 2,600 arthritis patients with osteoarthritis and Rheumatoid arthritis.[21] The results were shocking: Almost 80% of respondents *have used, used, or considered using* CBD products. Of those using CBD products, 94% reported using them for pain relief.

The results of the survey on CBD products by the National Arthritis Foundation Survey (2022) showed:
- 67% with improved physical functioning
- 30% improved morning stiffness
- 30% improved fatigue
- 71% better improvement in their sleep
- 67% less depression

In response to the uptick and results, the National Arthritis Foundation released a statement concerning the use of CBD, saying:

1. CBD *may help* with arthritis-related symptoms, such as pain, insomnia, and anxiety, but *there have been no rigorous clinical studies* on people with arthritis to confirm this.

2. While no significant safety issues have been found with CBD when taken in *moderate doses*, potential drug interactions have been identified.

3. CBD should never be used to replace disease-modifying drugs that help prevent permanent joint damage in inflammatory types of arthritis.
4. CBD use should be discussed with your doctor in advance, with follow-up evaluations every three months or so, as would be done for any new treatment.
5. There are no established clinical guidelines to inform usage.

If you're considering trying CBD oil for your RA symptoms, speak with your doctor first. Despite its relative safety, CBD can interact with your other medications, including antihypertensives, warfarin, antidepressants, anxiolytics, and anti-epileptic drugs.

> ○ **PROTIP**
>
> **CBD products do not replace your RA treatment (DMARDs or biologics).**

So, what about dosage? There's no universal dosage recommendation, so I suggest starting with a minimal amount and monitoring your body's reaction. Over time, you can slowly increase your dosage. Always stick to or below the dosage recommended in the product you've purchased.

CBD oil won't replace your current RA medication or treatment plan. However, it could potentially minimize your need for drugs, especially NSAIDs or opioids. It could also help with your pain, sleep, and fatigue.

I hope you, like many of my patients, finish this section with a sense of hope. Try some of these natural remedies that do work and are safe for RA, and stay away from so-called remedies that don't yield results and can cause dangerous health effects.

Important things to consider before buying CBD products

- Closely read product labels and check reviews.
- Do your research, and consult your doctor.
- Identify the manufacturer or distributor and research them as well.
- Verify product identity and cannabinoid content.
- Check quantity, batch/lot numbers, and the product's expiration date
- Follow instructions for use, dosing, and appropriate storage.

CHAPTER 11

THE POWER OF COMMUNITY

I love going for walks in the morning; I'm lucky enough to live near a park, and each day, I walk around my block and into the grassy area, noticing the groups of students congregating on benches, hunched over books. I smile at the people laughing at the dog park and those jogging with one another on the path surrounding the park. I embark on this walk daily, partially because movement helps me think in the morning and partially because I love seeing people genuinely enjoying one another without any underlying motivation.

For thousands of years, humans have lived in community with one another. Communities helped our ancestors meet and succeed in their challenges, share food, care for their children, and build shelters. Later on in our ancestry, these communities served as the basis through which we developed moral systems, as parents and children learned and taught one another the difference between right and wrong.[1] Expanding social networks were the basis for the world's earliest civilizations; building social networks encouraged our survival, paving the way for civilization as we know it.

Humans inherently require each other's physical, emotional, moral, and psychological support. We're prosocial beings designed to depend on, protect, and have empathy for one another.

You aren't alone: In fact, you're among a million people struggling with RA in the United States, with millions more abroad.

Loneliness On the Rise

Unfortunately, social connection is declining; conversely, loneliness is rising. Starting in the early 2000s, social isolation, companionship, and social engagement with friends and family started declining. Fast forward to 2022, according to the U.S. Surgeon General's report, only 39% of Americans are feeling deeply connected with those around them.[2]

Why is this important to note?

Well, over the last 30 years, loneliness has been shown to have a disastrous impact on our health. Many studies showed that social isolation and loneliness increase the number of hospitalizations, ER visits, and suicides. Loneliness is also the cause of increased incidences of chronic diseases like heart disease, diabetes, depression, and anxiety.

Social isolation's effects on health
• 29% increase in the risk of heart disease
• 36% increased risk for hypertension
• 32% increased risk of stroke
• 68% increased risk for hospitalization
• 57% increase in ER visits
• 50% increased risk of dementia
• 39% increase in the risk of early death

These aren't the only statistics on the importance of social connection: Studies show that those who are more socially connected to their family, friends, and community are happier, healthier, and live longer than those who aren't as connected. [3] For example, those who are socially isolated are 75% percent more likely to experience a rapid decline in their health to the point of death. It's a little dramatic but no less correct! These odds point to our innate need for social connection.

Social connection is a significant concern for everyone, particularly older adults or those aged 50 and older. As we age, it's common for our social networks to get smaller due to retirement, mobility issues, and losing loved ones. This can cause significant health issues like the ones we discussed above.

Stay Connected: RA & Loneliness

Struggling with RA, or any chronic illness for that matter, can be an isolating, lonely experience.[4] Eileen Davidson, a writer struggling with RA, states in an essay written for a national RA support website that since her diagnosis, she "[finds] it challenging to connect with the people I once knew, causing me to turn inward. Every aspect of my life has been altered by chronic illness — from my interests, daily routines, dreams, and even my spirit." And, most prominently, "out of all the changes brought on by chronic illness, loneliness, and social isolation are the most painful."[5]

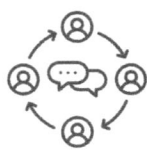

Her words echo my patients' sentiments: Many self-isolate because those around them don't understand what they're experiencing. Some have trouble "communicating the severity of their symptoms," and others attempt "to hide their symptoms from others."[6] As a result, sometimes "symptoms [are] the catalyst for the breakdown of relationships." One study examined nearly 160 RA patients and found that disease activity and disability significantly and reciprocally (positively and negatively) impacted patients' relationships. Close relationships seemed to suffer or benefit the most.[7]

RA significantly impacts patients' mood and social connectedness, causing a sense of helplessness and anger.[8] All of this can increase disease activity, causing more pain and fatigue, which, in turn, causes less social interaction. Furthermore, a lack of social connection strongly influences pain.[7] Another study illustrated that participants who lacked social connection experienced more pain. In other words, a lack of social connection causes emotional pain, aggravating physical pain.[9] So, while isolation can be tempting for RA patients, it only aggravates your symptoms.

> **COVID-19 & Community**
>
> One study looked specifically at RA patients' social well-being in the context of the recent COVID-19 pandemic and found that, throughout the epidemic, social well-being decreased for those with RA. Isolation seemed to cause fear in these patients and a lost sense of self-identity.

Social connection aids healing: RA patients who find openness and understanding in their significant others are more inclined to seek medical help.[6] Furthermore, a recent study examined social connection and health-related outcomes, looking closely at self-efficacy, empowerment, and mood. Researchers separated participants into two groups: one that had access to a secret Facebook group that offered patients RA-related discussion topics for 26 weeks and another group that didn't have access to this platform. The findings were clear: Self-efficacy and knowledge about their disease increased significantly for those with access to the Facebook community, resulting in better health and fewer symptoms.[10]

To summarize, stronger relationships lessen disease activity, or swollen joints, fatigue, and pain, and more robust disease activity positively impacts a patient's sense of social connection.

Release Yourself From the Loneliness Trap

 When I use the term "relationship", I'm not solely referring to your romantic relationships. Your friendships and other connections are relationships, too! Relationships are those in which you have an interpersonal link with the other person, and the two of you mutually influence the other's thoughts, feelings, and actions.

Good relationships are usually healthy and warm. You can tell the other person anything and feel a great deal of trust in them. You know that, despite occasional anger and frustration, the two of you will figure out your disagreements. Good relationships are full of respect and mutual understanding, not shame or blame.

Think about the relationships in your life. Which do you characterize as "good," and why?

These are the relationships you need to prioritize: These individuals will understand when you're not up to something or need extra time or help with your symptoms. In a good relationship, the other members won't say that they, "Don't get it" or that, "You try harder." Instead, they'll offer you space to share your pain, and they'll listen intently.

It's not about the number of relationships you have; instead, the quality of these relationships matters.

Don't isolate yourself from others. Though isolation might be tempting, doing so will only worsen how you're feeling and won't benefit you, your disease, or your pain. Instead, look for ways to be in community with those around you. Activities like dinner with friends or family, involvement in community and religious groups, and travel have been shown to improve your overall health and well-being and contribute to successful aging and disease management for arthritis patients.[11]

> **How do you become more connected?**
> 1. Chat with a stranger on the street. This practice boosts mood!
> 2. Over the next seven days, focus on making one new social connection daily. Spark up a conversation with someone while

> taking public transportation, ask a coworker about their day, or chat with the barista at the coffee shop.
> 3. Strengthen the relationships you already have. For a week, spend one-hour daily reconnecting with someone you care about (e.g., a friend who's moved far away or a family member you haven't spoken to in a while)

You aren't alone: In fact, you're among a million people struggling with RA in the United States, with millions more abroad. With the help of the internet, you can connect with these people and find a welcoming community of individuals who uniquely understand your pain.

I have built a community on social media: I have a Facebook group called Rheumatoid arthritis Warriors, and we have more than 20,000 members and counting! Through this group, I offer resources based on science and help people connect and support each other in their journey. We maintain a positive attitude and find solutions. Additionally, the National Arthritis Foundation offers local chapters to give a sense of community and empower people to fight arthritis.

> **To build stronger, positive relationships**
> ACTION STEPS
> 1. Choose someone you want to seek a deeper connection with (a family member or a friend).
> 2. Pick an activity you can do with this person regularly (e.g., walking together, weekly lunches or coffee dates, or regular phone calls).
> 3. Schedule a time to talk to this person about your plans and connect with them more often. Tell them how important this is for you.
> 4. Determine a consistent time for the two of you to meet weekly or monthly.

Get Connected

RA can be a lonely disease. As Davidson mentioned in her essay, many RA patients feel like no one will understand or that they won't be accommodated if they ask for help. The issue is this: RA, and the loneliness that accompanies it, significantly exacerbates your pain, inflammation, and fatigue. Not only that, but loneliness leaves you prey to many unwelcome conditions that negatively impact your health.

While you might feel alone right now, you're far from it. As I've mentioned throughout this book, you're in a vast group of over a million people struggling with the same thing you are. With the help of the internet, you can connect with these people and find a welcoming community of individuals who uniquely understand your pain.

CHAPTER 12

BECOME THE CEO OF YOUR RA

Jon, a patient of mine, struggled with RA for many years. But he was a fighter—he came to appointments early, asked plenty of questions, and maintained a positive attitude. Over the years, Jon incorporated everything I've explained in this book: He adopted a new, high-fiber, low-sugar diet, developed his exercise routine, incorporated mindfulness and meditation, and began sleeping more. Over time, and with continuous effort, Jon's symptoms improved; swelling in his hands had subsided, his morning stiffness was negligible, and his pain was gone.

Recently, I entered the exam room, eager to greet Jon. He looked excited, like he had some news for me; as his doctor, who'd seen his remarkable progress, I waited in anticipation.

He said, almost giddily, "So, you know that I was out of the country, right?"

I nodded, still waiting.

"Well," he began. "I'd decided to take on a big challenge and climb Mt. Kilimanjaro!"

I paused, almost in shock, and smiled wide. He continued, "I signed up for the six-day Lemosho route of hiking and camping. You know that I'm regularly active, but I was still so nervous about my RA on the climb. Rarely am I active all day—let alone for six days straight!"

I gave Jon a much-deserved hug. "I'm so happy for you," I said. "How was it?"

"The climb was intense," he said with a chuckle. "We hiked six-eight hours daily, but I reached the summit! On that day, we hiked for 12 hours, and it turns out I had a much harder time breathing at high elevations than I did dealing with my RA. One night, my hands became pretty numb after gripping the hiking poles all day, but they loosened up by the morning. And after the hike, my whole body was wrecked. But after two days, I recovered and went off on a safari!"

Nothing compared to the smile I had on my face when Jon told me the news. I told him that I was writing a book about RA and that I planned to share all of my knowledge about the holistic, comprehensive approach I'd discussed with him over the years. He was so excited and offered to share his story to help inspire others struggling with the same disease he suffers from.

I was beyond proud of him and accepted his offer. I'm also beyond proud of the changes possible when my patients have the agency to change their habits.

The changes you make are for **you**, your RA, and your mental health. Jon serves as an emblem for my patients, illustrating that, with some effort, remission and a great life are ultimately possible!

RA and Your Health-Related Quality of Life

Unfortunately, RA can have a profound impact on a patient's health-related quality of life (abbreviated as HRQoL). HRQol is a scientific measure that determines a person's overall health and well-being and how a disease or condition may impact it. A recent study asked RA patients like yourself,

"Do you feel that RA is impacting your life?" and "To what extent is RA altering your habits?"

As I'm sure you, an RA patient, can attest to, the study found that RA seriously influences a patient's quality of life and general well-being.[1] If left untreated, RA comes with serious issues that negatively impact a patient's physical functioning; these are often accompanied by nearly more severe problems with a patient's social well-being and mental health. To make matters worse, traditional treatments don't work for all patients, leaving 30-40% without relief from painful symptoms.

Luckily, all of the dietary changes, supplements, mindfulness techniques, exercises, sleep, and natural remedies discussed in this book can help you regain control over your RA. Studies confirm this again and again: Patients with RA who prioritize community, eat well, exercise, and manage their stress levels feel significantly better, with less pain and inflammation, than those who don't.[2]

The Blue Zone Lifestyle: Coming Full Circle

In his famous book, *The Blue Zones Solution: Eating and Living Like the World's Healthiest People* Dan Buettner described a phenomenon we see in some regions of the world: People living in Icaria, Greece, Loma Linda, California, Sardinia, Italy, Okinawa, Japan, and Nicoya, Costa Rica, live longer, happier and healthier lives.[3,4] Buettner describes these as 'blue zones.' Individuals living in 'blue zones' enjoy drastically lower rates of chronic disease and longer life expectancy.

So—why is this the case?

Diet is one of the primary contributors to blue zone residents' higher quality of life. Those living in blue zones tend to consume higher quantities of fruits, vegetables, whole grains, legumes, and nuts, with a lower-than-average consumption of meat and dairy products. They drink alcohol moderately and only as a part of social or cultural traditions. This dietary pattern might sound a little familiar: Much of the research available on the Mediterranean diet (see Chapter 5 for more information) comes from research on blue zones.

A calorie deficit may contribute to the longevity of those living in blue zones. For example, before the 1960s, citizens of Okinawa, Japan, often lived in a calorie deficit, eating fewer calories than their bodies required, which improved their longevity.[5] Today, citizens of Okinawa follow an 80% rule, meaning that they stop eating when they're 80% full as opposed to 100% (check out Chapter 5 for more information about incorporating healthier food options into your life.)

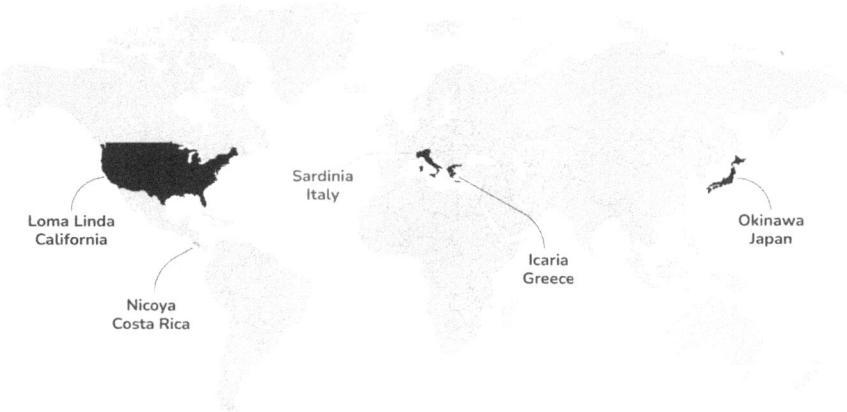

Figure 6. The word map and the blue zones distribution.

More than that, people living in blue zones engage in daily movements, like walking to a friend's house, grocery store, or work. They often perform regular manual labor, like gardening or cleaning (check out Chapter 8 for more helpful ways to get you moving more). Instead of scheduling exercise, which can be stressful, they try to move more every day, contributing to overall feelings of satisfaction.[6] In fact, even a short walk can help people live longer; recent studies show that the number of steps we take per day directly correlates with lifespan.[7]

The habits of blue zone inhabitants drastically differ from those of many living in the U.S. For example, those living in blue zones get plenty of sleep, often taking naps throughout the day if they get tired. Unlike U.S. residents, individuals living in blue zones don't "work through lunch," skip meals, or watch TV to fall asleep. Rather, they go to sleep when the sun goes down and wake when the sun rises. As we discussed in Chapter 9, eight hours of sleep are crucial, and research shows that inadequate sleep causes multiple chronic conditions and shortens lifespans.[8]

Social engagement is vital to these blue zones' culture: Strong social connections and regular interactions with those around them, especially family members, are part of everyday life. Living with and near family gives those living in blue zones a sense of purpose, allowing them to maintain a positive outlook on their lives.[9] Contrastingly, those living in the U.S. rarely live in a community with friends or family. Purpose is linked to lifespan, and living near family and friends is a powerful way to improve yours (don't be afraid to look at Chapter 11 for more tips on social engagement).

Most Americans live a life opposite of those living in blue zones: Our diets are animal-based, not plant-based. A 2010 report from the National Cancer Institute found that three out of four Americans don't eat a single piece of fruit on any given day, and few reach their minimums for fiber (see Chapters 4 and 5 for more information on fiber).[10] Most Americans don't meet their daily minimums for exercise, and our rigorous work schedule doesn't allow for naps or rest throughout the day. Along with that, many Americans are lonelier than ever, as we discussed in Chapter 11.

Those with RA must take particular note of this information: If your RA isn't adequately treated, you can potentially experience a shorter lifespan. While the exact numbers are unclear, studies show that RA shortens a patient's lifespan between 15% and 20%.[11] As we discussed in Chapter 3, RA patients are at an increased risk of developing other chronic diseases, like heart and lung disease, obesity, and even increased risk for cancers.

> **How to live a blue-zone lifestyle**
> - Eat a diet rich in plant-based foods. Consume minimal meat products while eating more fish.
> - Limit alcohol consumption to a glass a day maximum.
> - Try to move, not exercise. Build movement into your day, and walk as much as you can.
> - Incorporate rest and relaxation into your life. Meditate and practice mindfulness.
> - Sleep for eight to nine hours every day.
> - Be social, meet your family and friends often, and avoid toxic relationships.

All of the tips we discussed in this chapter combined bolster the results researchers see in blue zones—eating **a colorful, plant-based diet**, incorporating **meditation and mindfulness**, **moving more**, getting **plenty of sleep**, **relaxing,** and **spending time with loved ones**—all of these are ways in which you can get started with a blue zone lifestyle while still managing your RA.

Reclaim Your Future With RA

Throughout this book, we've discussed the inner workings of RA, what it is and what it isn't, and how clinicians like myself can help you get started with a treatment plan. Then, we talked about how—and why—you should clean up your diet and introduced RA-friendly foods to help you fight inflammation, mitigate pain, and reduce uncomfortable morning stiffness. We noted some essential supplements you can take to support your treatment plan. We introduced mindfulness and meditation as stress-reduction techniques to help you gain better control of your disease. We reviewed the importance of exercise, moving, and sleep, covering some vital sleep-boosting measures, and noted some crucial tools to help you get moving again like my patient Jon. Finally, we reviewed some helpful (and not-so-helpful) remedies to help you cope with your disease and the importance of connecting with others to support your treatment process.

Years of steady scientific research bolstered all the information we covered. Furthermore, the patient stories I've collected through my 20 years of medical practice solidify my claims. In other words, I've seen these astounding results and transformations firsthand.

The goal is to thrive, not merely survive.

By following these steps and consistently using these tools, I can assure you that you'll achieve both physical and psychological benefits, including less pain, inflammation, stiffness, swelling, easy movement, satisfaction, and happiness.

While RA can be exhausting, debilitating, and costly, it doesn't necessarily have to be. I urge you, and anyone fighting this condition, to become the CEO of your RA. It's okay to be a little overwhelmed when you're diagnosed or living with RA at times, but I assure you, **you're much more than this disease.**

It's time to come full circle: Embrace the changes, shifts, and suggestions I've offered in this book. I guarantee you—like Jon, you'll thank me, and your body will thank you. You can, and will, take charge of your RA—you just need to know where to start, and that's with this book.

The benefits are clear, and the choice to change is yours. Make it today.

You can and will take charge of your RA—you need to know where to start, and that's with this book.

REFERENCES

Chapter 2. Understanding the Past to Improve the Present

[1]Entezami P, Fox DA, Clapham PJ, Chung KC. Historical perspective on the etiology of rheumatoid arthritis. *Hand Clin.* 2011 Feb;27(1):1-10. doi: 10.1016/j.hcl.2010.09.006. PMID: 21176794; PMCID: PMC3119866.

[2]Simple Task Campaign https://rheumatology.org/patient-advocacy-awareness-simple-tasks

Chapter 3. Rheumatoid Arthritis 101

[1]Frisell T, Holmqvist M, Källberg H, Klareskog L, Alfredsson L, Askling J. Familial risks and heritability of rheumatoid arthritis: Role of rheumatoid factor/anti-citrullinated protein antibody status, number and type of affected relatives, sex, and age. *Arthritis Rheum.* 2013 Nov;65(11):2773-82. doi: 10.1002/art.38097. PMID: 23897126.

[2]Kovacs, W., Olsen, N. Sexual dimorphism of RA manifestations: genes, hormones and behavior. *Nat Rev Rheumatol* 7, 307–310 (2011). https://doi.org/10.1038/nrrheum.2010.231

[3]Harding AT, Heaton NS. The Impact of Estrogens and Their Receptors on Immunity and Inflammation during Infection. Cancers (Basel). 2022 Feb 12;14(4):909. doi: 10.3390/cancers14040909. PMID: 35205657; PMCID: PMC8870346.

[4]Talsania M, Scofield RH. Menopause and rheumatic disease. Rheum Dis Clin North Am. 2017 May;43(2):287-302. doi: 10.1016/j.rdc.2016.12.011. PMID: 28390570; PMCID: PMC5385852.

[5]Sammaritano LR, Bermas BL, Chakravarty EE, et al. 2020 American College of Rheumatology Guideline for the Management of Reproductive Health in Rheumatic and Musculoskeletal Diseases. *Arthritis Care & Research.* 2020;72(4):461-488. doi:https://doi.org/10.1002/acr.24130

[6]Qin B, Yang M, Fu H, Ma N, Wei T, Tang Q, Hu Z, Liang Y, Yang Z, Zhong R. Body mass index and the risk of rheumatoid arthritis: A systematic review and dose-response meta-analysis. *Arthritis Res Ther.* 2015 Mar 29;17(1):86. doi: 10.1186/s13075-015-0601-x. PMID: 25890172; PMCID: PMC4422605.

[7]Nezamoleslami S, Ghiasvand R, Feizi A, Salesi M, Pourmasoumi M. The relationship between dietary patterns and rheumatoid arthritis: a case–control study. *Nutrition & Metabolism.* 2020;17(1). doi:https://doi.org/10.1186/s12986-020-00502-7

[8]Sugiyama D, Nishimura K, Tamaki K, Tsuji G, Nakazawa T, Morinobu A, Kumagai S. Impact of smoking as a risk factor for developing rheumatoid arthritis: a meta-analysis

of observational studies. *Ann Rheum Dis.* 2010 Jan;69(1):70-81. doi: 10.1136/ard.2008.096487. PMID: 19174392.

[9]Alfredsson L, Klareskog L, Hedström AK. Influence of smoking on disease activity and quality of life in patients with rheumatoid arthritis: Results from a Swedish case-control study with longitudinal follow-up. *Arthritis Care Res (Hoboken).* 2023 Jun;75(6):1269-1277. doi: 10.1002/acr.25026. Epub 2023 Jan 16. PMID: 36149365.

[10]Lee YC, Agnew-Blais J, Malspeis S, Keyes K, Costenbader K, Kubzansky LD, Roberts AL, Koenen KC, Karlson EW. Post-Traumatic stress disorder and risk for incident rheumatoid arthritis. *Arthritis Care Res (Hoboken).* 2016 Mar;68(3):292-8. doi: 10.1002/acr.22683. PMID: 26239524; PMCID: PMC4740283.

[11]Baimukhamedov C, Barskova T, Matucci-Cerinic M. Arthritis after SARS-CoV-2 infection. *Lancet Rheumatol.* 2021 May;3(5):e324-e325. doi: 10.1016/S2665-9913(21)00067-9. Epub 2021 Mar 16. PMID: 33748780; PMCID: PMC7963449.

[12]Spagnoli LG, Bonanno E, Sangiorgi G, Mauriello A. Role of inflammation in atherosclerosis. *J Nucl Med.* 2007 Nov;48(11):1800-15. doi: 10.2967/jnumed.107.038661. Epub 2007 Oct 17. PMID: 17942804.

[13]Petri M, Elkhalifa M, Li J, Magder LS, Goldman DW. Hydroxychloroquine blood levels predict hydroxychloroquine retinopathy. *Arthritis & Rheumatology.* 2020;72(3):448-453. doi:https://doi.org/10.1002/art.41121

[14]Felson D. Defining remission in rheumatoid arthritis. *Ann Rheum Dis.* 2012 Apr;71 Suppl 2(0 2):i86-8. doi: 10.1136/annrheumdis-2011-200618. PMID: 22460146; PMCID: PMC3648878.

[15]Mease P, Charles-Schoeman C, Cohen S, Fallon L, Woolcott J, Yun H, Kremer J, Greenberg J, Malley W, Onofrei A, Kanik KS, Graham D, Wang C, Connell C, Valdez H, Hauben M, Hung E, Madsen A, Jones TV, Curtis JR. Incidence of venous and arterial thromboembolic events reported in the tofacitinib rheumatoid arthritis, psoriasis and psoriatic arthritis development programmes and from real-world data. Ann Rheum Dis. 2020 Nov;79(11):1400-1413. doi: 10.1136/annrheumdis-2019-216761. Epub 2020 Aug 5. PMID: 32759265; PMCID: PMC7569391.

[16]Ytterberg SR, Bhatt DL, Mikuls TR, Koch GG, Fleischmann R, Rivas JL, Germino R, Menon S, Sun Y, Wang C, Shapiro AB, Kanik KS, Connell CA; ORAL Surveillance Investigators. Cardiovascular and cancer risk with tofacitinib in rheumatoid arthritis. *N Engl J Med.* 2022 Jan 27;386(4):316-326. doi: 10.1056/NEJMoa2109927. PMID: 35081280.

[17]Bhandari S, Bhandari S, Bhandari S. Chimeric antigen receptor T cell therapy for the treatment of systemic rheumatic diseases: a comprehensive review of recent literature. *Ann Med Surg (Lond).* 2023 Jun 5;85(7):3512-3518. doi: 10.1097/MS9.0000000000000891. PMID: 37427200; PMCID: PMC10328598.

[18]Shimizu Y, Ntege EH, Azuma C, Uehara F, Toma T, Higa K, Yabiku H, Matsuura N, Inoue Y, Sunami H. Management of rheumatoid arthritis: Possibilities and challenges of mesenchymal stromal/stem cell-based therapies. *Cells.* 2023 Jul 21;12(14):1905. doi: 10.3390/cells12141905. PMID: 37508569; PMCID: PMC10378234.

Chapter 4. Trust Your Gut

[1] Sender R, Fuchs S, Milo R. Revised estimates for the number of human and bacteria cells in the body. *PLoS Biol.* 2016 Aug 19;14(8):e1002533. doi: 10.1371/journal.pbio.1002533. PMID: 27541692; PMCID: PMC4991899.

[2] Ferranti EP, Dunbar SB, Dunlop AL, Corwin EJ. 20 things you didn't know about the human gut microbiome. *The Journal of Cardiovascular Nursing.* 2014;29(6):479-481. doi:https://doi.org/10.1097/jcn.0000000000000166

[3] Harvard School of Public Health. The Microbiome. *The Nutrition Source.* Published September 4, 2019. https://www.hsph.harvard.edu/nutritionsource/microbiome/

[4] MD WB. *Fiber Fueled: The Plant-Based Gut Health Program for Losing Weight, Restoring Your Health, and Optimizing Your Microbiome.* Avery; 2020. Accessed April 10, 2024. https://www.amazon.com/Fiber-Fueled-Plant-Based-Optimizing-Microbiome/dp/059308456X

[5] Madison A, Kiecolt-Glaser JK. Stress, depression, diet, and the gut microbiome: human-bacteria interactions at the core of psychoneuroimmunology and nutrition. *Curr Opin Behav Sci.* 2019 Aug;28:105-110. doi: 10.1016/j.cobeha.2019.01.011. Epub 2019 Mar 25. PMID: 32395568; PMCID: PMC7213601.

[6] Gerritsen RJS, Band GPH. Breath of life: The respiratory vagal stimulation model of contemplative activity. *Front Hum Neurosci.* 2018 Oct 9;12:397. doi: 10.3389/fnhum.2018.00397. PMID: 30356789; PMCID: PMC6189422.

[7] Malesza IJ, Malesza M, Walkowiak J, Mussin N, Walkowiak D, Aringazina R, Bartkowiak-Wieczorek J, Mądry E. High-fat, western-style diet, systemic inflammation, and gut microbiome: A narrative review. *Cells.* 2021 Nov 14;10(11):3164. doi: 10.3390/cells10113164. PMID: 34831387; PMCID: PMC8619527.

[8] *Prescription drugs.* Health Policy Institute. https://hpi.georgetown.edu/rxdrugs/#:~:text=More%20than%20131%20million%20people

[9] Worby CJ, Olson BS, Dodson KW, Earl AM, Hultgren SJ. Establishing the role of the gut microbiome in susceptibility to recurrent urinary tract infections. *J Clin Invest.* 2022 Mar 1;132(5):e158497. doi: 10.1172/JCI158497. PMID: 35229729; PMCID: PMC8884912.

[10] Durack J, Lynch SV. The gut microbiome: Relationships with disease and opportunities for therapy. *The Journal of Experimental Medicine.* 2018;216(1):20-40. doi:https://doi.org/10.1084/jem.20180448

[11] Rosser EC, Mauri C. A clinical update on the significance of the gut microbiome in systemic autoimmunity. *J Autoimmun.* 2016 Nov;74:85-93. doi: 10.1016/j.jaut.2016.06.009. Epub 2016 Jul 29. PMID: 27481556.

[12] Chen Y, Chen L, Xing C, Deng G, Zeng F, Xie T, Gu L, Yang H. The risk of rheumatoid arthritis among patients with inflammatory bowel disease: a systematic review and meta-analysis. *BMC Gastroenterol.* 2020 Jun 17;20(1):192. doi: 10.1186/s12876-020-01339-3. PMID: 32552882; PMCID: PMC7301504.

[13] Kaur S, White S, Bartold M. Periodontal disease as a risk factor for rheumatoid arthritis: A systematic review. *JBI Libr Syst Rev.* 2012;10(42 Suppl):1-12. doi: 10.11124/jbisrir-2012-288. PMID: 27820156.

[14]Cariz J. *Gut bacteria can trigger rheumatoid arthritis, patient study suggests*. American Association for the Advancement of Science. Published 2022. https://www.aaas.org/news/gut-bacteria-can-trigger-rheumatoid-arthritis-patient-study-suggests

[15]Bodkhe R, Balakrishnan B, Taneja V. The role of microbiome in rheumatoid arthritis treatment. *Ther Adv Musculoskelet Dis*. 2019 Jul 30;11:1759720X19844632. doi: 10.1177/1759720X19844632. PMID: 31431810; PMCID: PMC6685117.

[16]Gupta, V.K., Cunningham, K.Y., Hur, B. et al. Gut microbial determinants of clinically important improvement in patients with rheumatoid arthritis. *Genome Med* 13, 149 (2021). https://doi.org/10.1186/s13073-021-00957-0

[17]Zaragoza-García O, Castro-Alarcón N, Pérez-Rubio G, Guzmán-Guzmán IP. DMARDs-gut microbiome feedback: Implications in the response to therapy. *Biomolecules*. 2020 Oct 24;10(11):1479. doi: 10.3390/biom10111479. PMID: 33114390; PMCID: PMC7692063.

[18]Zhao T, Wei Y, Zhu Y, Xie Z, Hai Q, Li Z, Qin D. Gut microbiome and rheumatoid arthritis: From pathogenesis to novel therapeutic opportunities. *Front Immunol*. 2022 Sep 8;13:1007165. doi: 10.3389/fimmu.2022.1007165. PMID: 36159786; PMCID: PMC9499173.

[19]Coras R, Martino C, Gauglitz JM, Cedola F, Tripathi A, Jarmusch AK, Alharthi M, Fernandez-Bustamante M, Agustin-Perez M, Singh A, Choi SI, Rivera T, Nguyen K, Shekhtman T, Holt T, Lee S, Golshan S, Dorrestein PC, Knight R, Guma M. Baseline microbiome and metabolome are associated with response to ITIS diet in an exploratory trial in patients with rheumatoid arthritis. *Clin Transl Med*. 2022 Jul;12(7):e959. doi: 10.1002/ctm2.959. PMID: 35802808; PMCID: PMC9269999.

[20]Chriswell ME, Lefferts AR, Clay MR, Hsu AR, Seifert J, Feser ML, Rims C, Bloom MS, Bemis EA, Liu S, Maerz MD, Frank DN, Demoruelle MK, Deane KD, James EA, Buckner JH, Robinson WH, Holers VM, Kuhn KA. Clonal IgA and IgG autoantibodies from individuals at risk for rheumatoid arthritis identify an arthritogenic strain of Subdoligranulum. *Sci Transl Med*. 2022 Oct 26;14(668):eabn5166. doi: 10.1126/scitranslmed.abn5166. Epub 2022 Oct 26. PMID: 36288282; PMCID: PMC9804515.

[21]Bustamante MF, Agustín-Perez M, Cedola F, Coras R, Narasimhan R, Golshan S, Guma M. Design of an anti-inflammatory diet (ITIS diet) for patients with rheumatoid arthritis. *Contemp Clin Trials Commun*. 2020 Jan 21;17:100524. doi: 10.1016/j.conctc.2020.100524. PMID: 32025586; PMCID: PMC6997513.

Chapter 5. Nutrition 101: Detoxify, Heal, and Supercharge

[1]Faruque S, Tong J, Lacmanovic V, Agbonghae C, Minaya DM, Czaja K. The dose makes the poison: Sugar and obesity in the United States - a Review. *Pol J Food Nutr Sci*. 2019;69(3):219-233. doi: 10.31883/pjfns/110735. PMID: 31938015; PMCID: PMC6959843.

[2]O'Connor L, Imamura F, Brage S, Griffin SJ, Wareham NJ, Forouhi NG. Intakes and sources of dietary sugars and their association with metabolic and inflammatory markers. *Clin Nutr*. 2018 Aug;37(4):1313-1322. doi: 10.1016/j.clnu.2017.05.030. Epub 2017 Jun 17. PMID: 28711418; PMCID: PMC5999353.

[3]Malik VS, Hu FB. The role of sugar-sweetened beverages in the global epidemics of obesity and chronic diseases. *Nat Rev Endocrinol.* 2022 Apr;18(4):205-218. doi: 10.1038/s41574-021-00627-6. Epub 2022 Jan 21. PMID: 35064240; PMCID: PMC8778490.

[4]Chung M, Ma J, Patel K, Berger S, Lau J, Lichtenstein AH. Fructose, high-fructose corn syrup, sucrose, and nonalcoholic fatty liver disease or indexes of liver health: a systematic review and meta-analysis. *Am J Clin Nutr.* 2014 Sep;100(3):833-49. doi: 10.3945/ajcn.114.086314. Epub 2014 Aug 6. PMID: 25099546; PMCID: PMC4135494.

[5]Sigala DM, Hieronimus B, Medici V, Lee V, Nunez MV, Bremer AA, Cox CL, Price CA, Benyam Y, Abdelhafez Y, McGahan JP, Keim NL, Goran MI, Pacini G, Tura A, Sirlin CB, Chaudhari AJ, Havel PJ, Stanhope KL. The dose-response effects of consuming high fructose corn syrup-sweetened beverages on hepatic lipid content and insulin sensitivity in young adults. *Nutrients.* 2022 Apr 15;14(8):1648. doi: 10.3390/nu14081648. PMID: 35458210; PMCID: PMC9030734.

[6]Hu Y, Costenbader KH, Gao X, Al-Daabil M, Sparks JA, Solomon DH, Hu FB, Karlson EW, Lu B. Sugar-sweetened soda consumption and risk of developing rheumatoid arthritis in women. *Am J Clin Nutr.* 2014 Sep;100(3):959-67. doi: 10.3945/ajcn.114.086918. Epub 2014 Jul 16. PMID: 25030783; PMCID: PMC4135503.

[7]Tedeschi SK, Frits M, Cui J, Zhang ZZ, Mahmoud T, Iannaccone C, Lin TC, Yoshida K, Weinblatt ME, Shadick NA, Solomon DH. Diet and rheumatoid arthritis symptoms: Survey results from a rheumatoid arthritis registry. *Arthritis Care Res (Hoboken).* 2017 Dec;69(12):1920-1925. doi: 10.1002/acr.23225. PMID: 28217907; PMCID: PMC5563270.

[8]Li X, Alu A, Wei Y, Wei X, Luo M. The modulatory effect of high salt on immune cells and related diseases. *Cell Prolif.* 2022 Sep;55(9):e13250. doi: 10.1111/cpr.13250. Epub 2022 Jun 23. PMID: 35747936; PMCID: PMC9436908.

[9]Minamino H, Katsushima M, Hashimoto M, Fujita Y, Yoshida T, Ikeda K, Isomura N, Oguri Y, Yamamoto W, Watanabe R, Murakami K, Murata K, Nishitani K, Tanaka M, Ito H, Ohmura K, Matsuda S, Inagaki N, Morinobu A. Urinary sodium-to-potassium ratio associates with hypertension and current disease activity in patients with rheumatoid arthritis: a cross-sectional study. *Arthritis Res Ther.* 2021 Mar 27;23(1):96. doi: 10.1186/s13075-021-02479-x. PMID: 33773587; PMCID: PMC8004419.

[10]Hall KD, Ayuketah A, Brychta R, Cai H, Cassimatis T, Chen KY, Chung ST, Costa E, Courville A, Darcey V, Fletcher LA, Forde CG, Gharib AM, Guo J, Howard R, Joseph PV, McGehee S, Ouwerkerk R, Raisinger K, Rozga I, Stagliano M, Walter M, Walter PJ, Yang S, Zhou M. Ultra-processed diets cause excess calorie intake and weight gain: An inpatient randomized controlled trial of ad libitum food intake. *Cell Metab.* 2019 Jul 2;30(1):67-77.e3. doi: 10.1016/j.cmet.2019.05.008. Epub 2019 May 16. Erratum in: Cell Metab. 2019 Jul 2;30(1):226. Erratum in: Cell Metab. 2020 Oct 6;32(4):690. PMID: 31105044; PMCID: PMC7946062.

[11]La Cava A. Leptin in inflammation and autoimmunity. *Cytokine.* 2017 Oct;98:51-58. doi: 10.1016/j.cyto.2016.10.011. PMID: 27916613; PMCID: PMC5453851.

[12]Targońska-Stępniak B, Grzechnik K. Adiponectin and leptin as biomarkers of disease activity and metabolic disorders in rheumatoid arthritis patients. *J Inflamm Res.* 2022

Oct 13;15:5845-5855. doi: 10.2147/JIR.S380642. PMID: 36247076; PMCID: PMC9556275.

[13]Iikuni N, Lam QL, Lu L, Matarese G, La Cava A. Leptin and inflammation. *Curr Immunol Rev.* 2008 May 1;4(2):70-79. doi: 10.2174/157339508784325046. PMID: 20198122; PMCID: PMC2829991.

[14]Lu B, Driban JB, Duryea J, McAlindon T, Lapane KL, Eaton CB. Milk consumption and progression of medial tibiofemoral knee osteoarthritis: data from the Osteoarthritis Initiative. *Arthritis Care Res (Hoboken).* 2014 Jun;66(6):802-9. doi: 10.1002/acr.22297. PMID: 24706620; PMCID: PMC4201042.

[15]Sundström B, Ljung L, Di Giuseppe D. Consumption of meat and dairy products is not associated with the risk for rheumatoid arthritis among women: A population-based cohort study. *Nutrients.* 2019 Nov 19;11(11):2825. doi: 10.3390/nu11112825. PMID: 31752273; PMCID: PMC6893662.

[16]Warjri SB, Ete T, Beyong T, Barman B, Lynrah KG, Nobin H, Perme O. Coeliac disease with rheumatoid arthritis: An unusual association. *Gastroenterology Res.* 2015 Feb;8(1):167-168. doi: 10.14740/gr641w. Epub 2015 Feb 14. PMID: 27785291; PMCID: PMC5051177.

[17]Guagnano MT, D'Angelo C, Caniglia D, Di Giovanni P, Celletti E, Sabatini E, Speranza L, Bucci M, Cipollone F, Paganelli R. Improvement of inflammation and pain after three months' exclusion diet in rheumatoid arthritis patients. *Nutrients.* 2021 Oct 9;13(10):3535. doi: 10.3390/nu13103535. PMID: 34684536; PMCID: PMC8539601.

[18]Iablokov V, Sydora BC, Foshaug R, Meddings J, Driedger D, Churchill T, Fedorak RN. Naturally occurring glycoalkaloids in potatoes aggravate intestinal inflammation in two mouse models of inflammatory bowel disease. *Dig Dis Sci.* 2010 Nov;55(11):3078-85. doi: 10.1007/s10620-010-1158-9. Epub 2010 Mar 3. PMID: 20198430.

[19]Joe's Garage. 11 coffee drinking statistics you should know & what it means for you. Joe's Garage Coffee. Published January 18, 2022. https://joesgaragecoffee.com/blog/coffee-drinking-statistics/ https://ard.bmj.com/content/60/Suppl_1/A459.1

[20]Asoudeh F, Dashti F, Jayedi A, Hemmati A, Fadel A, Mohammadi H. Caffeine, coffee, tea and risk of rheumatoid arthritis: Systematic review and dose-response meta-analysis of prospective cohort studies. *Front Nutr.* 2022 Feb 10;9:822557. doi: 10.3389/fnut.2022.822557. PMID: 35223954; PMCID: PMC8866764.

[21]Karlson EW, Mandl LA, Aweh GN, Grodstein F. Coffee consumption and risk of rheumatoid arthritis. *Arthritis Rheum.* 2003 Nov;48(11):3055-60. doi: 10.1002/art.11306. PMID: 14613266.

[22]Silke CM, Murphy MS, Busteed S, Murphy TB, Phelan M, Molloy MG. FRI0034 Does heavy caffeine ingestion affect the efficacy of methotrexate. *Annals of the Rheumatic Diseases.* 2001;60(Suppl 1):A459-A459. doi:https://doi.org/10.1136/annrheumdis-2001.1163

[23]Benito-Garcia E, Heller JE, Chibnik LB, Maher NE, Matthews HM, Bilics JA, Weinblatt ME, Shadick NA. Dietary caffeine intake does not affect methotrexate efficacy in patients with rheumatoid arthritis. *J Rheumatol.* 2006 Jul;33(7):1275-81. PMID: 16821266.

²⁴He J, Zhang P, Shen L, Niu L, Tan Y, Chen L, Zhao Y, Bai L, Hao X, Li X, Zhang S, Zhu L. Short-Chain fatty acids and their association with signaling pathways in inflammation, glucose and lipid metabolism. *Int J Mol Sci.* 2020 Sep 2;21(17):6356. doi: 10.3390/ijms21176356. PMID: 32887215; PMCID: PMC7503625.

²⁵Nagpal R, Wang S, Ahmadi S, Hayes J, Gagliano J, Subashchandrabose S, Kitzman DW, Becton T, Read R, Yadav H. Human-origin probiotic cocktail increases short-chain fatty acid production via modulation of mice and human gut microbiome. *Sci Rep.* 2018 Aug 23;8(1):12649. doi: 10.1038/s41598-018-30114-4. PMID: 30139941; PMCID: PMC6107516.

²⁶Quagliani D, Felt-Gunderson P. Closing america's fiber intake gap: Communication strategies from a food and fiber summit. *Am J Lifestyle Med.* 2016 Jul 7;11(1):80-85. doi: 10.1177/1559827615588079. PMID: 30202317; PMCID: PMC6124841.

²⁷Häger J, Bang H, Hagen M, Frech M, Träger P, Sokolova MV, Steffen U, Tascilar K, Sarter K, Schett G, Rech J, Zaiss MM. The role of dietary fiber in rheumatoid arthritis patients: A feasibility study. *Nutrients.* 2019 Oct 7;11(10):2392. doi: 10.3390/nu11102392. PMID: 31591345; PMCID: PMC6836071.

²⁸Shin SA, Joo BJ, Lee JS, Ryu G, Han M, Kim WY, Park HH, Lee JH, Lee CS. Phytochemicals as anti-inflammatory agents in animal models of prevalent inflammatory diseases. *Molecules.* 2020 Dec 15;25(24):5932. doi: 10.3390/molecules25245932. PMID: 33333788; PMCID: PMC7765227.

²⁹Zhu F, Du B, Xu B. Anti-inflammatory effects of phytochemicals from fruits, vegetables, and food legumes: A review. *Crit Rev Food Sci Nutr.* 2018 May 24;58(8):1260-1270. doi: 10.1080/10408398.2016.1251390. Epub 2017 Jun 12. PMID: 28605204.

³⁰Schell J, Scofield RH, Barrett JR, Kurien BT, Betts N, Lyons TJ, Zhao YD, Basu A. Strawberries improve pain and inflammation in obese adults with radiographic evidence of knee osteoarthritis. *Nutrients.* 2017 Aug 28;9(9):949. doi: 10.3390/nu9090949. PMID: 28846633; PMCID: PMC5622709.

³¹Sobolev AP, Ciampa A, Ingallina C, Mannina L, Capitani D, Ernesti I, Maggi E, Businaro R, Del Ben M, Engel P, Giusti AM, Donini LM, Pinto A. Blueberry-based meals for obese patients with metabolic syndrome: A multidisciplinary metabolomic pilot study. *Metabolites.* 2019 Jul 10;9(7):138. doi: 10.3390/metabo9070138. PMID: 31295937; PMCID: PMC6680695.

³²Ghavipour M, Sotoudeh G, Tavakoli E, Mowla K, Hasanzadeh J, Mazloom Z. Pomegranate extract alleviates disease activity and some blood biomarkers of inflammation and oxidative stress in Rheumatoid Arthritis patients. *Eur J Clin Nutr.* 2017 Jan;71(1):92-96. doi: 10.1038/ejcn.2016.151. Epub 2016 Aug 31. PMID: 27577177.

³³Müller S, März R, Schmolz M, Drewelow B, Eschmann K, Meiser P. Placebo-controlled randomized clinical trial on the immunomodulating activities of low- and high-dose bromelain after oral administration - new evidence on the antiinflammatory mode of action of bromelain. *Phytother Res.* 2013 Feb;27(2):199-204. doi: 10.1002/ptr.4678. Epub 2012 Apr 20. PMID: 22517542.

³⁴Pandey S, Cabot PJ, Shaw PN, Hewavitharana AK. Anti-inflammatory and immunomodulatory properties of Carica papaya. *J Immunotoxicol.* 2016 Jul;13(4):590-602. doi: 10.3109/1547691X.2016.1149528. Epub 2016 Jul 14. PMID: 27416522.

[35]Zhu F, Du B, Xu B. Anti-inflammatory effects of phytochemicals from fruits, vegetables, and food legumes: A review. *Crit Rev Food Sci Nutr.* 2018 May 24;58(8):1260-1270. doi: 10.1080/10408398.2016.1251390. Epub 2017 Jun 12. PMID: 28605204.

[36]Nguyen HD, Oh H, Kim MS. An increased intake of nutrients, fruits, and green vegetables was negatively related to the risk of arthritis and osteoarthritis development in the aging population. *Nutr Res.* 2022 Mar;99:51-65. doi: 10.1016/j.nutres.2021.11.005. Epub 2021 Dec 29. PMID: 35093832.

[37]Saraf-Bank S, Esmaillzadeh A, Faghihimani E, Azadbakht L. Effect of non-soy legume consumption on inflammation and serum adiponectin levels among first-degree relatives of patients with diabetes: a randomized, crossover study. *Nutrition.* 2015 Mar;31(3):459-65. doi: 10.1016/j.nut.2014.09.015. Epub 2014 Oct 18. PMID: 25701335.

[38]Salehi-Abargouei A, Saraf-Bank S, Bellissimo N, Azadbakht L. Effects of non-soy legume consumption on C-reactive protein: a systematic review and meta-analysis. *Nutrition.* 2015 May;31(5):631-9. doi: 10.1016/j.nut.2014.10.018. Epub 2014 Nov 7. PMID: 25837205.

[39/44]Estruch R, Ros E, Salas-Salvadó J, Covas MI, Corella D, Arós F, Gómez-Gracia E, Ruiz-Gutiérrez V, Fiol M, Lapetra J, Lamuela-Raventos RM, Serra-Majem L, Pintó X, Basora J, Muñoz MA, Sorlí JV, Martínez JA, Fitó M, Gea A, Hernán MA, Martínez-González MA; PREDIMED Study Investigators. Primary Prevention of Cardiovascular Disease with a Mediterranean Diet Supplemented with Extra-Virgin Olive Oil or Nuts. *N Engl J Med.* 2018 Jun 21;378(25):e34. doi: 10.1056/NEJMoa1800389. Epub 2018 Jun 13. PMID: 29897866.

[40]Dai J, Miller AH, Bremner JD, Goldberg J, Jones L, Shallenberger L, Buckham R, Murrah NV, Veledar E, Wilson PW, Vaccarino V. Adherence to the mediterranean diet is inversely associated with circulating interleukin-6 among middle-aged men: a twin study. *Circulation.* 2008 Jan 15;117(2):169-75. doi: 10.1161/CIRCULATIONAHA.107.710699. Epub 2007 Dec 17. PMID: 18086924; PMCID: PMC3232063.

[41]Zamani B, Golkar HR, Farshbaf S, Emadi-Baygi M, Tajabadi-Ebrahimi M, Jafari P, Akhavan R, Taghizadeh M, Memarzadeh MR, Asemi Z. Clinical and metabolic response to probiotic supplementation in patients with rheumatoid arthritis: a randomized, double-blind, placebo-controlled trial. *Int J Rheum Dis.* 2016 Sep;19(9):869-79. doi: 10.1111/1756-185X.12888. Epub 2016 May 2. PMID: 27135916.

[42]Alipour B, Homayouni-Rad A, Vaghef-Mehrabany E, Sharif SK, Vaghef-Mehrabany L, Asghari-Jafarabadi M, Nakhjavani MR, Mohtadi-Nia J. Effects of Lactobacillus casei supplementation on disease activity and inflammatory cytokines in rheumatoid arthritis patients: a randomized double-blind clinical trial. *Int J Rheum Dis.* 2014 Jun;17(5):519-27. doi: 10.1111/1756-185X.12333. Epub 2014 Mar 27. PMID: 24673738.

[43]Abhari K, Shekarforoush SS, Hosseinzadeh S, Nazifi S, Sajedianfard J, Eskandari MH. The effects of orally administered Bacillus coagulans and inulin on prevention and progression of rheumatoid arthritis in rats. *Food Nutr Res.* 2016 Jul 15;60:30876. doi: 10.3402/fnr.v60.30876. PMID: 27427194; PMCID: PMC4947834.

⁴⁵Gioxari A, Kaliora AC, Marantidou F, Panagiotakos DP. Intake of ω-3 polyunsaturated fatty acids in patients with rheumatoid arthritis: A systematic review and meta-analysis. *Nutrition*. 2018 Jan;45:114-124.e4. doi: 10.1016/j.nut.2017.06.023. Epub 2017 Jul 8. PMID: 28965775.

⁴⁶Rimm EB, Appel LJ, Chiuve SE, et al. Seafood Long-Chain n-3 polyunsaturated fatty acids and cardiovascular disease: A science advisory from the American Heart Association. *Circulation*. 2018;138(1). doi:https://doi.org/10.1161/cir.0000000000000574

⁴⁷Makuch S, Więcek K, Woźniak M. The immunomodulatory and anti-inflammatory effect of curcumin on immune cell populations, cytokines, and in vivo models of rheumatoid arthritis. *Pharmaceuticals* (Basel). 2021 Apr 1;14(4):309. doi: 10.3390/ph14040309. PMID: 33915757; PMCID: PMC8065689.

⁴⁸Aryaeian N, Shahram F, Mahmoudi M, Tavakoli H, Yousefi B, Arablou T, Jafari Karegar S. The effect of ginger supplementation on some immunity and inflammation intermediate genes expression in patients with active Rheumatoid Arthritis. *Gene*. 2019 May 25;698:179-185. doi: 10.1016/j.gene.2019.01.048. Epub 2019 Mar 4. PMID: 30844477.

⁴⁹Altman RD, Marcussen KC. Effects of a ginger extract on knee pain in patients with osteoarthritis. *Arthritis Rheum*. 2001 Nov;44(11):2531-8. doi: 10.1002/1529-0131(200111)44:11<2531::aid-art433>3.0.co;2-j. PMID: 11710709.

⁵⁰Quesada I, de Paola M, Torres-Palazzolo C, Camargo A, Ferder L, Manucha W, Castro C. Effect of garlic's active constituents in inflammation, obesity and cardiovascular disease. *Curr Hypertens Rep*. 2020 Jan 10;22(1):6. doi: 10.1007/s11906-019-1009-9. PMID: 31925548.

⁵¹Xu C, Mathews AE, Rodrigues C, Eudy BJ, Rowe CA, O'Donoughue A, Percival SS. Aged garlic extract supplementation modifies inflammation and immunity of adults with obesity: A randomized, double-blind, placebo-controlled clinical trial. *Clin Nutr ESPEN*. 2018 Apr;24:148-155. doi: 10.1016/j.clnesp.2017.11.010. Epub 2018 Jan 3. PMID: 29576354.

⁵²Letarouilly JG, Sanchez P, Nguyen Y, Sigaux J, Czernichow S, Flipo RM, Sellam J, Daïen C. Efficacy of spice supplementation in rheumatoid arthritis: A Systematic Literature Review. *Nutrients*. 2020 Dec 11;12(12):3800. doi: 10.3390/nu12123800. PMID: 33322318; PMCID: PMC7764619.

⁵³Alghadir AH, Gabr SA, Al-Eisa ES. Green tea and exercise interventions as nondrug remedies in geriatric patients with rheumatoid arthritis. *J Phys Ther Sci*. 2016 Oct;28(10):2820-2829. doi: 10.1589/jpts.28.2820. Epub 2016 Oct 28. PMID: 27821943; PMCID: PMC5088134.

⁵⁴Kris-Etherton P, Eckel RH, Howard BV, St Jeor S, Bazzarre TL. Nutrition Committee Population Science Committee and Clinical Science Committee of the American Heart Association. AHA Science Advisory: Lyon Diet Heart Study. Benefits of a Mediterranean-style, National Cholesterol Education Program/American Heart Association Step I Dietary Pattern on Cardiovascular Disease. *Circulation*. 2001 Apr 3;103(13):1823-5. doi: 10.1161/01.cir.103.13.1823. PMID: 11282918.

⁵⁵Johansson K, Askling J, Alfredsson L, Di Giuseppe D; EIRA study group. Mediterranean diet and risk of rheumatoid arthritis: a population-based case-control study. *Arthritis*

Res Ther. 2018 Aug 9;20(1):175. doi: 10.1186/s13075-018-1680-2. PMID: 30092814; PMCID: PMC6085628.

[56]Petre A. The Vegan Diet — A complete guide for beginners. Healthline. Published May 11, 2022. https://www.healthline.com/nutrition/vegan-diet-guide#other-benefits

[57]Craig WJ. Health effects of vegan diets. *Am J Clin Nutr.* 2009 May;89(5):1627S-1633S. doi: 10.3945/ajcn.2009.26736N. Epub 2009 Mar 11. PMID: 19279075.

[58]Tuso P, Ismail M, Ha B, Bartolotto C. Nutritional update for physicians: Plant-based diets. *The Permanente Journal.* 2013;17(2):61-66. doi:https://doi.org/10.7812/tpp/12-085

[59]Landry MJ, Ward CP, Cunanan KM, et al. Cardiometabolic effects of omnivorous vs vegan diets in identical twins: A randomized clinical trial. *JAMA Netw Open.* 2023;6(11):e2344457. doi:10.1001/jamanetworkopen.2023.44457

[60]Nenonen MT, Helve TA, Rauma AL, Hänninen OO. Uncooked, lactobacilli-rich, vegan food and rheumatoid arthritis. *Br J Rheumatol.* 1998 Mar;37(3):274-81. doi: 10.1093/rheumatology/37.3.274. PMID: 9566667.

[61]McDougall J, Bruce B, Spiller G, Westerdahl J, McDougall M. Effects of a very low-fat, vegan diet in subjects with rheumatoid arthritis. *J Altern Complement Med.* 2002 Feb;8(1):71-5. doi: 10.1089/107555302753507195. PMID: 11890437.

[62]Rondanelli M, Perdoni F, Peroni G, Caporali R, Gasparri C, Riva A, Petrangolini G, Faliva MA, Infantino V, Naso M, Perna S, Rigon C. Ideal food pyramid for patients with rheumatoid arthritis: A narrative review. *Clin Nutr.* 2021 Mar;40(3):661-689. doi: 10.1016/j.clnu.2020.08.020. Epub 2020 Sep 2. PMID: 32928578.

Chapter 6. The Not-So Bitter Pills

[1]Rosell M, Wesley AM, Rydin K, Klareskog L, Alfredsson L; EIRA study group. Dietary fish and fish oil and the risk of rheumatoid arthritis. *Epidemiology.* 2009 Nov;20(6):896-901. doi: 10.1097/EDE.0b013e3181b5f0ce. PMID: 19730266.

[2]Senftleber NK, Nielsen SM, Andersen JR, Bliddal H, Tarp S, Lauritzen L, Furst DE, Suarez-Almazor ME, Lyddiatt A, Christensen R. Marine oil supplements for arthritis pain: A systematic review and meta-analysis of randomized trials. *Nutrients.* 2017 Jan 6;9(1):42. doi: 10.3390/nu9010042. PMID: 28067815; PMCID: PMC5295086.

[3]Proudman SM, James MJ, Spargo LD, Metcalf RG, Sullivan TR, Rischmueller M, Flabouris K, Wechalekar MD, Lee AT, Cleland LG. Fish oil in recent onset rheumatoid arthritis: a randomised, double-blind controlled trial within algorithm-based drug use. *Ann Rheum Dis.* 2015 Jan;74(1):89-95. doi: 10.1136/annrheumdis-2013-204145. Epub 2013 Sep 30. PMID: 24081439.

[4]Maroon JC, Bost JW. Omega-3 fatty acids (fish oil) as an anti-inflammatory: an alternative to nonsteroidal anti-inflammatory drugs for discogenic pain. *Surg Neurol.* 2006 Apr;65(4):326-31. doi: 10.1016/j.surneu.2005.10.023. PMID: 16531187.

[5]Chandran B, Goel A. A randomized, pilot study to assess the efficacy and safety of curcumin in patients with active rheumatoid arthritis. *Phytother Res.* 2012 Nov;26(11):1719-25. doi: 10.1002/ptr.4639. Epub 2012 Mar 9. PMID: 22407780.

[6]Amalraj A, Varma K, Jacob J, Divya C, Kunnumakkara AB, Stohs SJ, Gopi S. A novel highly bioavailable curcumin formulation improves symptoms and diagnostic indicators

in rheumatoid arthritis patients: A randomized, double-blind, placebo-controlled, two-dose, three-arm, and parallel-group study. *J Med Food.* 2017 Oct;20(10):1022-1030. doi: 10.1089/jmf.2017.3930. Epub 2017 Aug 29. PMID: 28850308.

[7] Bagherniya M, Darand M, Askari G, Guest PC, Sathyapalan T, Sahebkar A. The clinical use of curcumin for the treatment of rheumatoid arthritis: A systematic review of clinical trials. *Adv Exp Med Biol.* 2021;1291:251-263. doi: 10.1007/978-3-030-56153-6_15. PMID: 34331695.

[8] Daily JW, Yang M, Park S. Efficacy of turmeric extracts and curcumin for alleviating the symptoms of joint arthritis: A systematic review and meta-analysis of randomized clinical trials. *J Med Food.* 2016 Aug;19(8):717-29. doi: 10.1089/jmf.2016.3705. PMID: 27533649; PMCID: PMC5003001.

[9] Vaghef-Mehrabany E, Alipour B, Homayouni-Rad A, Sharif SK, Asghari-Jafarabadi M, Zavvari S. Probiotic supplementation improves inflammatory status in patients with rheumatoid arthritis. *Nutrition.* 2014 Apr;30(4):430-5. doi: 10.1016/j.nut.2013.09.007. Epub 2013 Dec 17. PMID: 24355439.

[10] Kostoglou-Athanassiou I, Athanassiou P, Lyraki A, Raftakis I, Antoniadis C. Vitamin D and rheumatoid arthritis. *Ther Adv Endocrinol Metab.* 2012 Dec;3(6):181-7. doi: 10.1177/2042018812471070. PMID: 23323190; PMCID: PMC3539179.

[11] Manson JE, Cook NR, Lee IM, Christen W, Bassuk SS, Mora S, Gibson H, Gordon D, Copeland T, D'Agostino D, Friedenberg G, Ridge C, Bubes V, Giovannucci EL, Willett WC, Buring JE; VITAL Research Group. Vitamin D supplements and prevention of cancer and cardiovascular disease. *N Engl J Med.* 2019 Jan 3;380(1):33-44. doi: 10.1056/NEJMoa1809944. Epub 2018 Nov 10. PMID: 30415629; PMCID: PMC6425757.

[12] Tice JA, Halalau A, Burke H. Vitamin D Does Not Prevent Cancer or Cardiovascular Disease: The VITAL Trial : Manson JE, Cook NR, Lee IM, Christen W, Bassuk SS, Mora S, Gibson H, Gordon D, Copeland T, D'Agostino D, Friedenberg G, Ridge C, Bubes V, Giovannucci EL, Willett WC, Buring JE (2019) Vitamin D supplements and prevention of cancer and cardiovascular disease. N Engl J Med 380 (1):33-44. *J Gen Intern Med.* 2020 Aug 12. doi: 10.1007/s11606-020-05648-x. Epub ahead of print. PMID: 32789616.

[13] Merlino LA, Curtis J, Mikuls TR, Cerhan JR, Criswell LA, Saag KG; Iowa Women's Health Study. Vitamin D intake is inversely associated with rheumatoid arthritis: results from the Iowa Women's Health Study. *Arthritis Rheum.* 2004 Jan;50(1):72-7. doi: 10.1002/art.11434. PMID: 14730601.

[14] Meena N, Singh Chawla SP, Garg R, Batta A, Kaur S. Assessment of Vitamin D in rheumatoid arthritis and its correlation with disease activity. *J Nat Sci Biol Med.* 2018 Jan-Jun;9(1):54-58. doi: 10.4103/jnsbm.JNSBM_128_17. PMID: 29456394; PMCID: PMC5812075.

[15] Li Y, Yao J, Han C, et al. Quercetin, inflammation and immunity. *Nutrients.* 2016;8(3):167. doi:https://doi.org/10.3390/nu8030167

[16] Javadi F, Ahmadzadeh A, Eghtesadi S, Aryaeian N, Zabihiyeganeh M, Rahimi Foroushani A, Jazayeri S. The effect of quercetin on inflammatory factors and clinical symptoms in women with rheumatoid arthritis: A double-blind, randomized controlled trial. *J Am*

Coll Nutr. 2017 Jan;36(1):9-15. doi: 10.1080/07315724.2016.1140093. Epub 2016 Oct 6. PMID: 27710596.

[17]Ghavipour, M., Sotoudeh, G., Tavakoli, E. *et al.* Pomegranate extract alleviates disease activity and some blood biomarkers of inflammation and oxidative stress in Rheumatoid Arthritis patients. *Eur J Clin Nutr* 71, 92–96 (2017). https://doi.org/10.1038/ejcn.2016.151

[18]Xu C, Mathews AE, Rodrigues C, Eudy BJ, Rowe CA, O'Donoughue A, Percival SS. Aged garlic extract supplementation modifies inflammation and immunity of adults with obesity: A randomized, double-blind, placebo-controlled clinical trial. *Clin Nutr ESPEN.* 2018 Apr;24:148-155. doi: 10.1016/j.clnesp.2017.11.010. Epub 2018 Jan 3. PMID: 29576354.

[19]Helli B, Shahi MM, Mowla K, Jalali MT, Haghighian HK. A randomized, triple-blind, placebo-controlled clinical trial, evaluating the sesamin supplement effects on proteolytic enzymes, inflammatory markers, and clinical indices in women with rheumatoid arthritis. *Phytother Res.* 2019 Sep;33(9):2421-2428. doi: 10.1002/ptr.6433. Epub 2019 Jul 15. PMID: 31309643.

[20]Abdollahzad H, Aghdashi MA, Asghari Jafarabadi M, Alipour B. Effects of coenzyme q10 supplementation on inflammatory cytokines (TNF-α, IL-6) and oxidative stress in rheumatoid arthritis patients: A randomized controlled trial. *Arch Med Res.* 2015 Oct;46(7):527-33. doi: 10.1016/j.arcmed.2015.08.006. Epub 2015 Sep 3. PMID: 26342738.

[21]Aryaeian N, Shahram F, Mahmoudi M, Tavakoli H, Yousefi B, Arablou T, Jafari Karegar S. The effect of ginger supplementation on some immunity and inflammation intermediate genes expression in patients with active Rheumatoid Arthritis. *Gene.* 2019 May 25;698:179-185. doi: 10.1016/j.gene.2019.01.048. Epub 2019 Mar 4. PMID: 30844477.

[22]Kumar R, Singh S, Saksena AK, Pal R, Jaiswal R, Kumar R. Effect of boswellia serrata extract on acute inflammatory parameters and tumor necrosis factor-α in complete freund's adjuvant-induced animal model of rheumatoid arthritis. *Int J Appl Basic Med Res.* 2019 Apr-Jun;9(2):100-106. doi: 10.4103/ijabmr.IJABMR_248_18. PMID: 31041173; PMCID: PMC6477955.

Chapter 7. It's Not In Your Head: Stress, RA, and Healing

[1]Gordon E, Chauvin R, Van A, et al. A mind-body interface alternates with effector-specific regions in motor corte. Europe PMC. Published 2022. Accessed April 11, 2024. https://europepmc.org/article/ppr/ppr563687

[2]Liu YZ, Wang YX, Jiang CL. Inflammation: The common pathway of stress-related diseases. *Front Hum Neurosci.* 2017 Jun 20;11:316. doi: 10.3389/fnhum.2017.00316. PMID: 28676747; PMCID: PMC5476783.

[3]Littrell J. The mind-body connection: not just a theory anymore. *Soc Work Health Care.* 2008;46(4):17-37. doi: 10.1300/j010v46n04_02. PMID: 18589562.

[4]Lee YC, Agnew-Blais J, Malspeis S, Keyes K, Costenbader K, Kubzansky LD, Roberts AL, Koenen KC, Karlson EW. Post-traumatic stress disorder and risk for incident rheumatoid arthritis. *Arthritis Care Res (Hoboken).* 2016 Mar;68(3):292-8. doi: 10.1002/acr.22683. PMID: 26239524; PMCID: PMC4740283.

[5]Polinski KJ, Bemis EA, Feser M, Seifert J, Demoruelle MK, Striebich CC, Brake S, O'Dell JR, Mikuls TR, Weisman MH, Gregersen PK, Keating RM, Buckner J, Nicassio P, Holers VM, Deane KD, Norris JM. Perceived stress and inflammatory arthritis: A prospective investigation in the studies of the etiologies of rheumatoid arthritis cohort. *Arthritis Care Res (Hoboken)*. 2020 Dec;72(12):1766-1771. doi: 10.1002/acr.24085. Epub 2020 Nov 6. PMID: 31600025; PMCID: PMC7145743.

[6]De Brouwer SJ, Kraaimaat FW, Sweep FC, Creemers MC, Radstake TR, van Laarhoven AI, van Riel PL, Evers AW. Experimental stress in inflammatory rheumatic diseases: a review of psychophysiological stress responses. *Arthritis Res Ther*. 2010;12(3):R89. doi: 10.1186/ar3016. Epub 2010 May 17. PMID: 20478029; PMCID: PMC2911873.

[7]Edwards RR, Wasan AD, Bingham CO 3rd, Bathon J, Haythornthwaite JA, Smith MT, Page GG. Enhanced reactivity to pain in patients with rheumatoid arthritis. *Arthritis Res Ther*. 2009;11(3):R61. doi: 10.1186/ar2684. Epub 2009 May 4. PMID: 19413909; PMCID: PMC2714104.

[8]Niazi AK, Niazi SK. Mindfulness-based stress reduction: a non-pharmacological approach for chronic illnesses. *N Am J Med Sci*. 2011 Jan;3(1):20-3. doi: 10.4297/najms.2011.320. PMID: 22540058; PMCID: PMC3336928.

[9]DiRenzo D, Crespo-Bosque M, Gould N, Finan P, Nanavati J, Bingham CO 3rd. Systematic review and meta-analysis: Mindfulness-based interventions for rheumatoid arthritis. *Curr Rheumatol Rep*. 2018 Oct 18;20(12):75. doi: 10.1007/s11926-018-0787-4. PMID: 30338418; PMCID: PMC6233984.

[10]Lee AC, Harvey WF, Price LL, Morgan LPK, Morgan NL, Wang C. Mindfulness is associated with psychological health and moderates pain in knee osteoarthritis. *Osteoarthritis Cartilage*. 2017 Jun;25(6):824-831. doi: 10.1016/j.joca.2016.06.017. Epub 2016 Jun 24. PMID: 27349461; PMCID: PMC5183521.

[11]Majeed MH, Ali AA, Sudak DM. Mindfulness-based interventions for chronic pain: Evidence and applications. *Asian J Psychiatr*. 2018 Feb;32:79-83. doi: 10.1016/j.ajp.2017.11.025. Epub 2017 Dec 5. PMID: 29220782.

[12]*Meditation and mindfulness: What you need to know*. NCCIH. Published June 2022. https://www.nccih.nih.gov/health/meditation-and-mindfulness-what-you-need-to-know

[13]Rod K. Observing the effects of mindfulness-based meditation on anxiety and depression in chronic pain patients. *Psychiatr Danub*. 2015 Sep;27 Suppl 1:S209-11. PMID: 26417764.

[14]Slagter L, Demyttenaere K, Verschueren P, De Cock D. The effect of meditation, mindfulness, and yoga in patients with rheumatoid arthritis. *Journal of Personalized Medicine*. 2022;12(11):1905. doi:https://doi.org/10.3390/jpm12111905

[15]Gerszberg C. *Why your out-breath is connected to your well-being*. Mindful. Published September 9, 2021. https://www.mindful.org/why-your-breath-is-connected-to-your-well-being/

[16]Magnon, V., Dutheil, F. & Vallet, G.T. Benefits from one session of deep and slow breathing on vagal tone and anxiety in young and older adults. *Sci Rep* 11, 19267 (2021).

[17]Koopman FA, Chavan SS, Miljko S, Grazio S, Sokolovic S, Schuurman PR, Mehta AD, Levine YA, Faltys M, Zitnik R, Tracey KJ, Tak PP. Vagus nerve stimulation inhibits cytokine production and attenuates disease severity in rheumatoid arthritis. *Proc Natl Acad Sci U S A*. 2016 Jul 19;113(29):8284-9. doi: 10.1073/pnas.1605635113. Epub 2016 Jul 5. PMID: 27382171; PMCID: PMC4961187.

[18]Courties A, Berenbaum F, Sellam J. Vagus nerve stimulation in musculoskeletal diseases. *Joint Bone Spine*. 2021 May;88(3):105149.

[19]https://reset-ra.study/

[20]Koo M, Algoe SB, Wilson TD, Gilbert DT. It's a wonderful life: mentally subtracting positive events improves people's affective states, contrary to their affective forecasts. *J Pers Soc Psychol*. 2008 Nov;95(5):1217-24. doi: 10.1037/a0013316. PMID: 18954203; PMCID: PMC2746912.

[21]Emmons RA, McCullough ME. Counting blessings versus burdens: an experimental investigation of gratitude and subjective well-being in daily life. *J Pers Soc Psychol*. 2003 Feb;84(2):377-89. doi: 10.1037//0022-3514.84.2.377. PMID: 12585811.

[22]Jose, P. E., Lim, B. T., & Bryant, F. B. (2012). Does savoring increase happiness? A daily diary study. *The Journal of Positive Psychology*, 7(3), 176–187.

Gordon EM, Chauvin RJ, Van AN, Rajesh A, Nielsen A, Newbold DJ, Lynch CJ, Seider NA, Krimmel SR, Scheidter KM, Monk J, Miller RL, Metoki A, Montez DF, Zheng A, Elbau I, Madison T, Nishino T, Myers MJ, Kaplan S, Badke D'Andrea C, Demeter DV, Feigelis M, Ramirez JSB, Xu T, Barch DM, Smyser CD, Rogers CE, Zimmermann J, Botteron KN, Pruett JR, Willie JT, Brunner P, Shimony JS, Kay BP, Marek S, Norris SA, Gratton C, Sylvester CM, Power JD, Liston C, Greene DJ, Roland JL, Petersen SE, Raichle ME, Laumann TO, Fair DA, Dosenbach NUF. A Somato-Cognitive Action Network alternates with effector regions in motor cortex. *Nature*. April 19, 2023.

Chapter 8. Motion is Lotion: How to Get Movin'

[1]Basso JC, Suzuki WA. The effects of acute exercise on mood, cognition, neurophysiology, and neurochemical pathways: A review. *Brain Plast*. 2017 Mar 28;2(2):127-152.

[2]Ruegsegger GN, Booth FW. Health benefits of exercise. *Cold Spring Harb Perspect Med*. 2018 Jul 2;8(7):a029694. doi: 10.1101/cshperspect.a029694. PMID: 28507196; PMCID: PMC6027933.

[3]Usmani D, Ganapathy K, Patel D, Saini A, Gupta J, Dixit S. The role of exercise in preventing chronic diseases: Current evidence and recommendations. *Georgian Med News*. 2023 Jun;(339):137-142. PMID: 37522789.

[4]Wender CLA, Manninen M, O'Connor PJ. The effect of chronic exercise on energy and fatigue states: A systematic review and meta-analysis of randomized trials. *Front Psychol*. 2022 Jun 3;13:907637. doi: 10.3389/fpsyg.2022.907637. PMID: 35726269; PMCID: PMC9206544.

[5]García-Correa HR, Sánchez-Montoya LJ, Daza-Arana JE, Ordoñez-Mora LT. Aerobic physical exercise for pain intensity, aerobic capacity, and quality of life in patients with chronic pain: A systematic review and meta-analysis. *J Phys Act Health*. 2021 Aug 5;18(9):1126-1142.

[6]Myers J, Kokkinos P, Nyelin E. Physical activity, cardiorespiratory fitness, and the metabolic syndrome. *Nutrients.* 2019 Jul 19;11(7):1652.

[7]Metsios GS, Stavropoulos-Kalinoglou A, Kitas GD. The role of exercise in the management of rheumatoid arthritis. *Expert Rev Clin Immunol.* 2015;11(10):1121-30.

[8]Hu H, Xu A, Gao C, Wang Z, Wu X. The effect of physical exercise on rheumatoid arthritis: An overview of systematic reviews and meta-analysis. *J Adv Nurs.* 2021 Feb;77(2):506-522.

[9]Lange E, Kucharski D, Svedlund S, Svensson K, Bertholds G, Gjertsson I, Mannerkorpi K. Effects of aerobic and resistance exercise in older adults with rheumatoid arthritis: A randomized controlled trial. *Arthritis Care Res (Hoboken).* 2019 Jan;71(1):61-70.

[10]Mateen S, Moin S, Khan AQ, Zafar A, Fatima N, Shahzad S. Role of hydrotherapy in the amelioration of oxidant-antioxidant status in rheumatoid arthritis patients. *Int J Rheum Dis.* 2018 Oct;21(10):1822-1830.

[11]Eversden, L., Maggs, F., Nightingale, P. et al. A pragmatic randomised controlled trial of hydrotherapy and land exercises on overall well being and quality of life in rheumatoid arthritis. *BMC Musculoskelet Disord* 8, 23 (2007).

[12]Al-Qubaeissy KY, Fatoye FA, Goodwin PC, Yohannes AM. The effectiveness of hydrotherapy in the management of rheumatoid arthritis: a systematic review. *Musculoskeletal Care.* 2013 Mar;11(1):3-18.

Chapter 9. Get Some Rest: Sleep & RA

[1]Walker, M. (2018). *Why we sleep.* Penguin Books.

[2]Goel N, Rao H, Durmer JS, Dinges DF. Neurocognitive consequences of sleep deprivation. *Semin Neurol.* 2009 Sep;29(4):320-39.

[3]Irwin MR, Straub RH, Smith MT. Heat of the night: Sleep disturbance activates inflammatory mechanisms and induces pain in rheumatoid arthritis. *Nat Rev Rheumatol.* 2023 Sep;19(9):545-559.

[4]Kontodimopoulos N, Stamatopoulou E, Kletsas G, Kandili A. Disease activity and sleep quality in rheumatoid arthritis: a deeper look into the relationship. *Expert Rev Pharmacoecon Outcomes Res.* 2020 Dec;20(6):595-602.

[5]Stanciu I, Anderson J, Siebert S, Mackay D, Lyall DM. Associations of rheumatoid arthritis and rheumatoid factor with mental health, sleep and cognition characteristics in the UK Biobank. *Sci Rep.* 2022 Nov 18;12(1):19844.

[6]McBeth J, Dixon WG, Moore SM, Hellman B, James B, Kyle SD, Lunt M, Cordingley L, Yimer BB, Druce KL. Sleep disturbance and quality of life in rheumatoid arthritis: Prospective mHealth study. *J Med Internet Res.* 2022 Apr 22;24(4):e32825.

Chapter 10. Natural Remedies that Work (And Those That Don't)

[1]Zwolińska J, Gąsior M, Śnieżek E, Kwolek A. The use of magnetic fields in treatment of patients with rheumatoid arthritis. Review of the literature. *Reumatologia.* 2016;54(4):201-206. doi: 10.5114/reum.2016.62475. Epub 2016 Oct 5. PMID: 27826175; PMCID: PMC5090029.

[2]Richmond SJ, Gunadasa S, Bland M, MacPherson H (2013) Copper bracelets and magnetic wrist straps for rheumatoid arthritis – analgesic and anti-inflammatory effects: A randomised double-blind placebo controlled crossover trial. *PLoS ONE* 8(9): e71529.

[3]Tartari APS, Moreira FF, Pereira MCDS, Carraro E, Cidral-Filho FJ, Salgado AI, Kerppers II. Anti-inflammatory effect of ozone therapy in an experimental model of rheumatoid arthritis. *Inflammation*. 2020 Jun;43(3):985-993.

[4]Wang, C., Sun, W., Dalbeth, N. et al. Efficacy and safety of tart cherry supplementary citrate mixture on gout patients: a prospective, randomized, controlled study. *Arthritis Res Ther* 25, 164 (2023).

[5]Kashiuchi S, Miyazawa R, Nagata H, Shirai M, Shimizu M, Sone H, Kamiyama S. Effects of administration of glucosamine and chicken cartilage hydrolysate on rheumatoid arthritis in SKG mice. *Food Funct*. 2019 Aug 1;10(8):5008-5017.

[6]Lee JA, Son MJ, Choi J, Jun JH, Kim JI, Lee MS. Bee venom acupuncture for rheumatoid arthritis: a systematic review of randomised clinical trials. *BMJ Open*. 2014 Nov 7;4(11):e006140.

[7]Magnon V, Dutheil F, Vallet GT. Benefits from one session of deep and slow breathing on vagal tone and anxiety in young and older adults. *Scientific Reports*. 2021;11(1).

[8]Marsal S, Corominas H, de Agustín JJ, et al. Non-invasive vagus nerve stimulation for rheumatoid arthritis: a proof-of-concept study. *The Lancet Rheumatology*. 2021;3(4):e262-e269.

[9]Karagülle M, Kardeş S, Karagülle MZ. Long-term efficacy of spa therapy in patients with rheumatoid arthritis. *Rheumatology International*. 2018;38(3):353-362.

[10]Minden-Birkenmaier BA, Meadows MB, Cherukuri K, Smeltzer MP, Smith RA, Radic MZ, Bowlin GL. The effect of manuka honey on dHL-60 cytokine, chemokine, and matrix-degrading enzyme release under inflammatory conditions. *Med One*. 2019;4(2):e190005.

[11]Jahanban-Esfahlan R, Mehrzadi S, Reiter RJ, et al. Melatonin in regulation of inflammatory pathways in rheumatoid arthritis and osteoarthritis: involvement of circadian clock genes. *British Journal of Pharmacology*. 2017;175(16):3230-3238.

[12]Wróbel A, Szklarczyk J, Barańska I, Majda A, Jaworek J. Association between levels of serotonin, melatonin, cortisol and the clinical condition of patients with rheumatoid arthritis. *Rheumatol Int*. 2023 May;43(5):859-866. doi: 10.1007/s00296-023-05296-4. Epub 2023 Mar 13. PMID: 36912941; PMCID: PMC10073159.

[13]Oosterveld FGJ, Rasker JJ, Floors M, et al. Infrared sauna in patients with rheumatoid arthritis and ankylosing spondylitis. *Clinical Rheumatology*. 2008;28(1):29-34.

[14]Sprouse-Blum AS, Smith G, Sugai D, Parsa FD. Understanding endorphins and their importance in pain management. *Hawaii medical journal*. 2010;69(3):70-71. https://www.ncbi.nlm.nih.gov/pmc/articles/PMC3104618/

[15]CDC. *CBD: What You Need to Know*. CDC. Published August 8, 2022. https://www.cdc.gov/marijuana/featured-topics/CBD.

[16]Katz-Talmor D, Katz I, Porat-Katz BS, Shoenfeld Y. Cannabinoids for the treatment of rheumatic diseases — where do we stand? *Nature Reviews Rheumatology*. 2018;14(8):488-498.

[17]Jean-Gilles L, Braitch M, Latif ML, Aram J, Fahey AJ, Edwards LJ, Robins RA, Tanasescu R, Tighe PJ, Gran B, Showe LC, Alexander SP, Chapman V, Kendall DA, Constantinescu CS. Effects of pro-inflammatory cytokines on cannabinoid CB1 and CB2 receptors in immune cells. *Acta Physiol* (Oxf). 2015 May;214(1):63-74.

[18]Blake DR, Robson P, Ho M, Jubb RW, McCabe CS. Preliminary assessment of the efficacy, tolerability and safety of a cannabis-based medicine (Sativex) in the treatment of pain caused by rheumatoid arthritis. *Rheumatology*. 2005;45(1):50-52.

[19]Wipfler K, Simon TA, Katz P, Wolfe F, Michaud K. Increase in cannabis use among adults with rheumatic diseases: Results from a 2014⊠2019 US observational study. *Arthritis Care & Research*. Published online July 15, 2021.

[20]Frane N, Stapleton E, Iturriaga C, Ganz M, Rasquinha V, Duarte R. Cannabidiol as a treatment for arthritis and joint pain: an exploratory cross-sectional study. *Journal of Cannabis Research*. 2022;4(1).

[21]Patients Tell Us About CBD Use - News. Arthritis. Accessed April 12, 2024. https://www.arthritis.org/news/patients-tell-us-cbd-use

Chapter 11. The Power of Community

[1]Boyd R, Richerson PJ. Culture and the evolution of human cooperation. *Philos Trans R Soc Lond B Biol Sci*. 2009 Nov 12;364(1533):3281-8.

[2]Murthy V. *Our epidemic of loneliness and isolation*. 2023.

[3]Powell A. *How social isolation, loneliness can shorten your life*. Harvard Gazette. Published October 3, 2023.

[4]Park JYE, Howren AM, Davidson E, De Vera MA. Insights on mental health when living with rheumatoid arthritis: a descriptive qualitative study of threads on the Reddit website. *BMC Rheumatology*. 2020;4(1).

[5]Davidson E. *Confronting the challenges of loneliness and rheumatoid arthritis*. Creaky Joints. Published August 8, 2023. https://creakyjoints.org/about-arthritis/rheumatoid-arthritis/ra-patient-perspectives/loneliness-and-rheumatoid-arthritis/

[6]Tiwana R, Rowland J, Fincher M, Raza K, Stack RJ. Social interactions at the onset of rheumatoid arthritis and their influence on help-seeking behaviour: A qualitative exploration. *Br J Health Psychol*. 2015 Sep;20(3):648-61.

[7]Fitzpatrick R, Newman S, Lamb R, Shipley M. Social relationships and psychological well-being in rheumatoid arthritis. *Soc Sci Med*. 1988;27(4):399-403. doi: 10.1016/0277-9536(88)90275-4. PMID: 3175723.

[8]Lütze U, Archenholtz B. The impact of arthritis on daily life with the patient perspective in focus. *Scandinavian Journal of Caring Sciences*. 2007;21(1):64-70.

[9]Karos K, McParland JL, Bunzli S, Devan H, Hirsh A, Kapos FP, Keogh E, Moore D, Tracy LM, Ashton-James CE. The social threats of COVID-19 for people with chronic pain. Pain. 2020 Oct;161(10):2229-2235.

[10]Lopez-Olivo MA, Foreman JT, Leung C, Lin HY, Westrich-Robertson T, Hofstetter C, des Bordes JKA, Lyddiatt A, Leong A, Willcockson IU, Peterson SK, Suarez-Almazor ME. A randomized controlled trial evaluating the effects of social networking on chronic disease management in rheumatoid arthritis. *Semin Arthritis Rheum*. 2022 Oct;56:152072.

[11]Stevens-Ratchford, R., & Cebulak, B. J. (2005). Living well with arthritis: A study of engagement in social occupations and successful aging. *Physical & Occupational Therapy In Geriatrics*, 22(4), 31–52.

Ryan S, Campbell P, Paskins Z, Hider S, Manning F, Rule K, Brooks M, Hassell A. Exploring the physical, psychological and social well-being of people with rheumatoid arthritis during the coronavirus pandemic: a single-centre, longitudinal, qualitative interview study in the UK. *BMJ Open*. 2022 Jul 26;12(7):e056555.

Chapter 12. Become the CEO of Your RA

[1]Matcham F, Scott IC, Rayner L, Hotopf M, Kingsley GH, Norton S, Scott DL, Steer S. The impact of rheumatoid arthritis on quality-of-life assessed using the SF-36: a systematic review and meta-analysis. *Semin Arthritis Rheum*. 2014 Oct;44(2):123-30.

[2]Walrabenstein, W., van der Leeden, M., Weijs, P. et al. The effect of a multidisciplinary lifestyle program for patients with rheumatoid arthritis, an increased risk for rheumatoid arthritis or with metabolic syndrome-associated osteoarthritis: the "Plants for Joints" randomized controlled trial protocol. *Trials 22*, 715 (2021).

[3]Buettner D. *Blue Zones Solution, The: Eating and Living like the World's Healthiest People.* Reprint edition. National Geographic; 2017. Accessed April 12, 2024. https://www.amazon.com/Blue-Zones-Solution-Eating-Healthiest/dp/1426216556

[4]Buettner D, Skemp S. Blue Zones: Lessons From the World's Longest Lived. *Am J Lifestyle Med*. 2016 Jul 7;10(5):318-321.

[5]Willcox BJ, Willcox DC, Todoriki H, Fujiyoshi A, Yano K, He Q, Curb JD, Suzuki M. Caloric restriction, the traditional Okinawan diet, and healthy aging: the diet of the world's longest-lived people and its potential impact on morbidity and life span. *Ann N Y Acad Sci*. 2007 Oct;1114:434-55.

[6]Pes GM, Tolu F, Poulain M, Errigo A, Masala S, Pietrobelli A, Battistini NC, Maioli M. Lifestyle and nutrition related to male longevity in Sardinia: an ecological study. *Nutr Metab Cardiovasc Dis*. 2013 Mar;23(3):212-9.

[7]Lee IM, Paffenbarger RS Jr. Associations of light, moderate, and vigorous intensity physical activity with longevity. The Harvard Alumni Health Study. *Am J Epidemiol*. 2000 Feb 1;151(3):293-9.

[8]Shen X, Wu Y, Zhang D. Nighttime sleep duration, 24-hour sleep duration and risk of all-cause mortality among adults: a meta-analysis of prospective cohort studies. *Sci Rep*. 2016 Feb 22;6:21480.

[9]Hill PL, Turiano NA. Purpose in life as a predictor of mortality across adulthood. *Psychol Sci*. 2014 Jul;25(7):1482-6. doi: 10.1177/0956797614531799. Epub 2014 May 8. PMID: 24815612; PMCID: PMC4224996.

[10]CDC. *Majority of Americans not meeting recommendations for fruit and vegetable consumption.*; 2009. https://www.cdc.gov/media/pressrel/2009/r090929.htm

[11]Myllykangas-Luosujärvi R, Aho K, Kautiainen H, Isomäki H. Shortening of life span and causes of excess mortality in a population-based series of subjects with rheumatoid arthritis. *Clinical and Experimental Rheumatology*. 1995 Mar-Apr;13(2):149-153. PMID: 7656460.

PATIENT RESOURCES

Websites:
- https://rheumatologistoncall.com/
- https://www.arthritis.org/
- https://corigramescu.com

Youtube Channel: https://www.youtube.com/@rheumatologistoncall

RA Journal link: https://amzn.to/48rQE6n

Thriving with Arthritis Podcast https://podcasts.apple.com/us/podcast/thriving-with-arthritis/

Other books by Dr. Girnita " The Complete Gout Management and Nutrition Guide: Empowering Strategies for Better Health" Link: https://amzn.to/4dOkbtu

Connect with Dr. Diana Girnita

BLOG: https://rheumatologistoncall.com/blog/

Instagram: @rheumatologistoncall

Facebook: https://www.facebook.com/RheumatologistOncall

LinkedIn: https://www.linkedin.com/in/diana-girnita-md-phd-07b57810/

Facebook Group Rheumatoid arthritis Warriors https://www.facebook.com/groups/3685130571554200

Apps for Mindfulness:
- Headspace
- Calm
- Breathwrk

NOTE

NOTE

NOTE

PATIENT RESOURCES

www.ingramcontent.com/pod-product-compliance
Lightning Source LLC
Chambersburg PA
CBHW052028030426
42337CB00027B/4912